Recent Results in Cancer Research 124

Managing Editors
Ch. Herfarth, Heidelberg · H.-J. Senn, St. Gallen

Associate Editors
M. Baum, London · V. Diehl, Köln
F. Gutzwiller, Zürich · M. F. Rajewsky, Essen
M. Wannenmacher, Heidelberg

Founding Editor
R. Rentchnick, Geneva

Recent Results in Cancer Research

K. Höffken (Ed.)

Peptides in Oncology I

LH-RH Agonists and Antagonists

With 23 Figures and 11 Tables

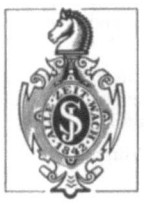

Springer-Verlag

Berlin Heidelberg New York
London Paris Tokyo
Hong Kong Barcelona
Budapest

Prof. Dr. K. Höffken
Innere Klinik und Poliklinik (Tumorforschung)
Universitätsklinikum Essen
Hufelandstraße 55, W-4300 Essen, FRG

ISBN-13: 978-88-470-2188-4   e-ISBN-13: 978-88-470-2186-0
DOI: 10.1007/978-88-470-2186-0

Library of Congress Cataloging-in-Publication Data
Peptides in oncology I : LH-RH agonists and antagonists / K. Höffken (ed.).
p cm. – (Recent results in cancer research ; v 124)   Includes bibliographical
references and index.

1. Luteinizing hormone releasing hormone – Agonists – Therapeutic use. 2. Luteinizing hormone releasing hormone – Antagonists – Therapeutic use. 3. Cancer – Hormone therapy. 4. Generative organs – Cancer – Hormone therapy. I. Höffken, K.
(Klaus), 1946– II. Title: Peptides in oncology 1. III. Title. Peptides in oncology one.
IV. Series   [DNLM: 1. Gonadorelin – antagonists & inhibitors. 2. Neoplasms –
drug therapy.   W1   RE106P   v. 124]   RC261.R35   vol. 124   [RC271.L87]
616.99′4 s – dc20   [616.99′4061]   DNLM/DLC   92-2203

© Springer-Verlag Berlin Heidelberg 1992
Softcover reprint of the hardcover 1st edition 1992

Typesetting, printing, binding: K. Triltsch, Graphischer Betrieb, Würzburg
65/3130-5 4 3 2 1 0 – Printed on acid-free paper

Preface

Hormonal treatment of malignant diseases has been used for quite some years now, and progress in this field is still being made at a steady pace. The detection of new endocrine feedback loops and the availability of new classes of hormonal agents made hormonal intervention with predictable outcome possible. Besides the intellectual challenge of modulating the hormone system, an important aspect of recent research on hormones and cancer is the reduction of treatment-related morbidity achieved with the new hormonal strategies. Thus, controlled intervention in the hypothalamic-gonadotropic axis is increasingly apt to replace surgical removal of the relevant glands, i.e., the pituitary gland or the gonads. In the same way as, for example, aromatase inhibitors are being used as a substitute for adrenalectomy.

The concept that secretion of hypothalamic gonadotropin-releasing hormone (GnRH), pituitary gonadotropins, and sex steroids are regulated via negative and positive feedback loops is based on the pioneering work of Hohlweg and Harris some 40 years ago.

In 1971, a breakthrough was achieved with the isolation, structural analysis, and synthesis of the luteinizing hormone releasing hormone (LH-RH), or GnRH as it is now more appropriately termed, since it provokes the secretion of both gonadotropins, LH and FSH, and since then the progress made in this area of research has been remarkable. Both agonists and antagonists of LH-RH have been synthesized and extensively studied in preclinical and clinical settings.

It soon became apparent that agonists of LH-RH are capable of inducing a hypogonadotropic gonadal insufficiency, thus clearing the way for the use of these substances in the treatment of hormone-sensitive neoplasms, classically prostate and breast cancer. Gonadal ablation in the treatment of these malignancies has a long history. Thus, it was both logical and scientifically appealing to replace the irreversible surgical procedures with medical therapy. Evidence has accumulated over the past years that LH-RH agonists can serve as "medical orchiectomy" in prostate cancer. As a logical consequence, the hypogonadotropic gonadal insufficiency induced by LH-RH agonists was investigated in patients with breast cancer. Here too it appears that "medical oophorectomy" can serve to replace the surgical procedure. In addition, ovarian and endometrical cancer have become targets for treatment with LH-RH agonists. These antineoplastic effects are obviously mediated both via hormonal feedback loops and by direct LH-RH binding sites. Furthermore, as benign neoplasms with estrogen-dependent growth, uterine leiomyomas can now be successfully treated with LH-RH agonists.

Finally, evidence has been accumulated over the past few years which suggests that LH-RH agonists alone or in combination with other peptides (e.g., somatostatin) are capable of transiently controlling the growth of pancreatic cancer in both preclinical and clinical settings. By contrast, LH-RH agonists were unable to induce responses in any of 31 patients suffering from hepatocellular carcinoma. It should be mentioned in this context that anecdotal observations exist on the successful treatment of gonadotropin-producing pituitary tumors.

Parallel to the development of a number of synthetic analogs of the native decapeptide LH-RH, progress has been made in investigations into the synthesis and applicability of the antagonists of LH-RH.

Scientific literature has rapidly accumulated over the past years in the field of peptides, i.e., hormones and growth factors, in oncologic treatment in general and of LH-RH in particular, and it appears timely to update the available knowledge. The first volume of *Peptides in Oncology* contains contributions from experts on LH-RH agonists and antagonists in oncology, dealing with mechanisms of action, clinical results of the treatment of prostate, breast, ovarian, endometrial, and pancreatic cancer, and benign uterine leiomyomas, and providing an overview of LH-RH antagonists.

This volume provides an update of the results achievable using LH-RH agonists and antagonists in oncology and indicates aspects of future basic and clinical research in the field. Clearly, the end result will be an optimum number of patients benefiting from these treatment modalities.

It is my privilege and pleasure to acknowledge the assistance of Mrs. G. Cönenberg as well as Mrs. S. Benko and Dr. T. Thiekötter from Springer-Verlag for the contribution of their expertise in the completion of this book.

Essen, January 1992   K. Höffken

Contents

List of Contributors *

---

* The addresses of the authors are given on the first page of each contribution.
[1] Page on which contribution begins.

Mechanisms of Action of LH-RH Agonists

Gonadotropin-Releasing Hormone: Physiological and Endocrinological Aspects

D. Klingmüller[1] and H. U. Schweikert[2]

[1] Abteilung Endokrinologie, Institut für Klinische Biochemie, Universität Bonn, Sigmund-Freud-Straße 25, W-5300 Bonn, FRG
[2] Medizinische Universitäts-Poliklinik, Wilhelmstraße 35, W-5300 Bonn, FRG

Biological processes are time dependent and mostly take the form of recurring cycles which are subject to active and inactive periods. Apparently, process of natural selection favored a cycle in which an organism was not required to function at maximum capacity all the time, but could transiently pause at distinct intervals (Bünning 1967). Many hormones are released episodically, the length of the episodes depending on the individual rhythms of the hormones. The spectrum of releasing frequencies is widely distributed; yearly, monthly, daily, and hourly rhythms are known. In the animal system, seasonal rutting is a well-known example, while in humans, examples include the female menstrual cycle, the circadian secretion of adrenocorticotropic hormone (ACTH), and the 1- to 2-h pulse secretion of gonadotropin-releasing hormone (GnRH).

GnRH secretion from the hypothalamus is particularly interesting, since the target organ of the hormone requires pulsating stimulation in order to activate its own secretion process. The pituitary gland can only be prompted into long-term secretion of gonadotropins when it receives pulsatile stimulation, that is, repeated stimulation at regular intervals. By contrast, continuous administration of GnRH or long-acting GnRH analogs suppresses gonadotropin secretion. Thus, GnRH has two different and opposing effects: stimulation and suppression of the pituitary-gonadal axis. GnRH is a decapeptide that is made up of ten amino acids with a molecular weight totaling 1181 daltons. The following chemical structure has been recognized: pGlu-His-Trp-Ser-Tyr-Gly-Leu-Arg-Pro-GlyNH$_2$. The serum half-life of GnRH is short and ranges between 2 and 9 min (Arimura et al. 1974; Jeffcoate et al. 1974, Miyachi et al. 1973; Pimstone et al. 1977). By substituting amino acids, the enzymatic breakdown can be delayed and the half-life prolonged. By substituting the original GnRH with the analog buserelin, which has D-Ser(t-Bu) in position 6, or with the analog [D-Trp^6]-GnRH, which has tryptophan in position 6, the degradation takes substantially longer than with natural GnRH. In this way, hormonal activity can be greatly prolonged.

Recent Results in Cancer Research, Vol. 124
© Springer-Verlag Berlin · Heidelberg 1992

A gene for GnRH has been isolated (Nikolics et al. 1985) that codes for a 56 amino acid protein. This so-called gonadotropin-releasing hormone-associated peptide (GAP) stimulates the secretion of luteinizing hormone (LH) and follicle-stimulating hormone (FSH). In addition, it inhibits the excretion of prolactin to a greater extent than dopamine.

The detailed regulation of GnRH-induced effects on the pituitary cells are still unclear. As far as we know today, GnRH binds to its receptor, and the signal transduction requires several intracellular messenger systems to induce gonadotropin secretion. The interaction of GnRH with its receptor activates the mobilization of calcium and, via a G protein, activates phospholipase C which metabolizes the polyphosphoinositides to inositol phosphates (Schrey 1985). The accumulation of calcium activates calmodulin, which appears to mediate the release of gonadotropins. Calcium in combination with diacylglycerol activates protein kinase C (Hirota et al. 1985), which appears to mediate the biosynthesis of gonadotropins.

GnRH is produced in the hypothalamus. From the area preoptica and the nucleus arcuatus in the mediobasal part of the hypothalamus, it travels via neurons to the median eminence, where it is released into the hypophysioportal circulation. The regulation of GnRH secretion is complex. Visual, olfactory, and tactile stimulants are processed in the cerebral cortex and sent as neural information to the hypothalamus. Here the signal is translated in to an endocrine message. As well as being prompted by exogenous stimuli, GnRH secretion can also be prompted by a variety of endogenous factors. Here the neurotransmitters noradrenaline, adrenaline, and serotonin are important, as are opioids and the hormones of the pituitary-gonadal axis, particularly gonadal steroids. Lastly, prostaglandins and calcium participate as intracellular transmitting agents in the release of GnRH. GnRH is transported via the pituitary portal vein system to the anterior pituitary lobe. There it stimulates the gonadotrophic cells to produce and secrete the gonadotropins LH and FSH.

In turn, LH stimulates the production and secretion of testosterone by the testicular Leydig cells, while FSH activates spermatogenesis and probably also the development of a secondary hormone, inhibin, in the Sertoli cells. Through chemical reactions, testosterone and inhibin are able to suppress the release of gonadotropins and thus their own secretion. For example, inhibin specifically suppresses the secretion of FSH, while testosterone suppresses the release of LH and FSH in that it decreases pituitary sensitivity to the GnRH secreted by the hypothalamus.

In this way, the hormones of the hypothalamic-pituitary-gonadal axis are regulated by a complex feedback system. Above and beyond this, the principal regulatory substance, GnRH, is responsible for inducing puberty. The hypothalamus probably secretes GnRH as a result of a decrease in sensitivity of the suppressing effect of the sex hormones (Gonadostat theory; Boyer et al. 1974). After transient episodes of GnRH secretion during the neonatal period and before the onset of puberty, the secretion of gonadotropin is low. A pulsatile pattern of secretion is not, or only to a small extent, present. During puberty, the oscillatory-like activity of the hypothalamus begins. This prompts the pulsatile secretion of GnRH which regulates the LH-FSH secretion of the pituitary gland. At first only nocturnally, increased pulsatile secretion of LH and FSH takes place. As puberty advances, the pattern of secretion continues with increasing amplitude during the whole day until adult hormone levels are reached. As a result the blood level of testosterone in men increases, and the development of secondary sex characteristics begins. The final step is then spermatogenesis. If this development does not take place as a result of insufficient GnRH secretion, hypogonadotropic hypogonadism results.

As mentioned above, GnRH is released via neurons of the hypothalamus into the portal vein system of the pituitary. The GnRH neurons are activated in a cyclic and synchronized fashion, so that pulsatile secretion of GnRH results. A complete separation of the mediobasal section of the hypothalamus from the rest of the central nervous system in oophorectomized rhesus monkeys had no effect on the pulsatile secretion of GnRH (Krey et al. 1975). Thus, it can be assumed that the pacemaker for the synchronized activity in monkeys, and probably also in humans, is located in this area of the hypothalamus. This was confirmed by studies of Wilson and coworkers. They found that characteristic increases in neuronal activity coincide with the pulsatile release of LH from the pituitary gland. This was recorded from electrodes chronically implanted in the medial basal region of the hypothalamus in rhesus monkeys (Wilson et al. 1983).

The pulsatile type of secretion is, as Knobil and his coworkers found in their investigations (Krey et al. 1975), the determining factor for the release of gonadotropins from the pituitary. They used rhesus monkeys which could no longer produce GnRH due to experimentally induced destruction of the hypothalamus. The animals were oophorectomized in order to eliminate the influence of sex hormones on the pituitary. The continuous presence of GnRH led at first to a marked increase in the release of LH and FSH. This was followed by a refractory phase, during which the pituitary could not be stimulated, and the secretion of gonadotropin was suppressed.

In contrast, with pulsatile stimulation the pituitary was prompted to secrete LH and FSH for several weeks (Fig. 1). Continuous stimulation of the pituitary in humans was first accomplished by Leyendecker et al. (1980) in women and by Hoffman and Crowley (1982) and our group, for example (Klingmüller et al. 1983), in men. In particular, it was possible in patients with Kallmann's syndrome, which is characterized by hypothalamic hypogonadism and anosmia, to induce puberty and spermatogenesis by subcutaneous administration of GnRH. In addition, spermatogenesis was maintained by means of intranasal administration of GnRH (Klingmüller et al. 1985).

In vitro, Smith and Vale (1981) were able to show that with pulsatile administration of GnRH, pituitary cells remained responsive to stimulation over a 24-h period. Continuous administration, on the other hand, led within 12 h to a rapid decrease in hormone secretion.

The precise mechanism of downregulation is still unclear. First, a decrease in GnRH receptors takes place. Secondly, receptor levels return to normal, and supranormal desensitization is further maintained by uncoupling of the

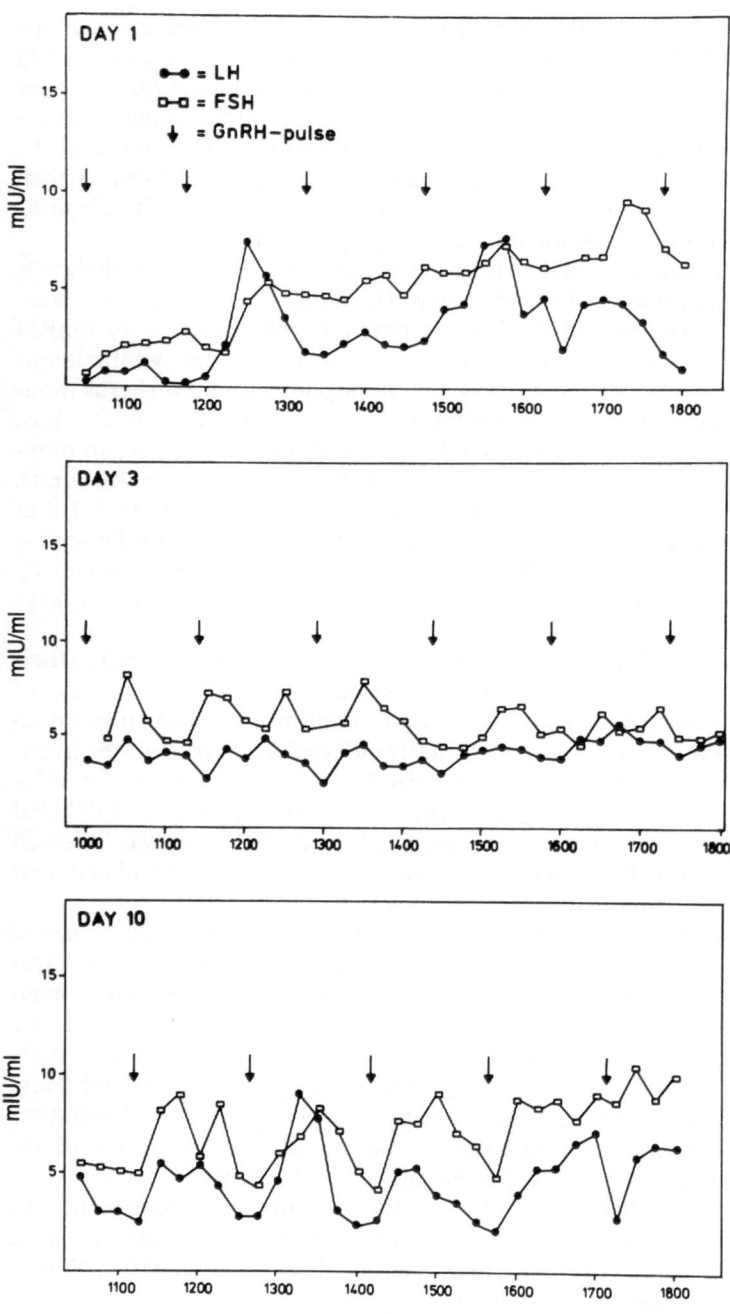

Fig. 1. Secretion profiles of LH and FSH in a patient suffering from Kallmann's syndrome on days 1, 3, and 10 of treatment with 5 µg GnRH every 90 min

receptor from their intracellular mediators. In contrast to the GnRH agonists, GnRH antagonists suppress gonadotropin secretion immediately by competitive blockade of the GnRH receptor (Conn and Crowley 1991).

In summary, the pituitary gland responds with long-term gonadotropin secretion only when it receives pulsatile stimulation with hypothalamic GnRH. This physiological pattern of release has substantial corollaries for the therapeutic use of GnRH. Exogenous GnRH can only prompt long-term secretion of LH and FSH from the anterior pituitary gland if the latter receives intermittent stimulation every 90–120 min (Santen and Bardin 1973). Continuous stimulation of the pituitary GnRH receptors with GnRH agonists or blockade of the receptor by GnRH antagonists has the opposite effect, i.e., suppression of gonadotropin secretion. This gives rise to a number of interesting therapeutic possibilities as outlined below.

Clinical Applications of GnRH and Its Analogues

1. Stimulation of pituitary and gonadal function
   GnRH test
   Cryptorchidism
   Induction of ovulation in hypothalamic amenorrhea
   Induction of puberty in delayed puberty and hypogonadism due to inadequate GnRH secretion
2. Inhibition of pituitary and gonadal function
   Pubertas praecox
   Endometriosis
   Uterine fibroids
   Contraception
   Adjuvant treatment in sexual-steroid-sensitive tumors of breast and prostate

References

Arimura A, Kastin AJ, Schally AV (1974) Immunoreactive LH-releasing hormone in plasma: midcycle elevation in women. J Clin Endocrinol Metab 38:510

Boyar RM, Rosenfeld RS, Kapen S, Finkelstein JW, Roffwarg HP, Weitzmann ED, Hellmann L (1974) Human puberty: simultaneous augmented secretion of luteinizing hormone and testosterone during sleep. J Clin Invest 54:609

Bünning E (1967) Gesetzmäßigkeiten der Chronobiologie. Verh Dtsch Ges Innere Med 73:887

Conn PM, Crowley WF (1991) Gonadotropin-releasing hormone and its analogues. N Engl J Med 324:93

Hirota K, Hirota T, Aquilera G, Catt KJ (1985) Hormone induced redistribution of calcium activated phospholipid-dependent protein kinase in pituitary gonadotrophs. J Biol Chem 260:3243

Hoffman AR, Crowley WF (1982) Induction of puberty in men by long-term pulsatile administration of low-dose gonadotropin-releasing hormone. N Engl J Med 307:1237

Jeffcoate SL, Greenwood RH, Holland DT (1974) Blood and urine clearance of luteinizing hormone releasing hormone in man measured by radioimmunoassay. J Endocrinol 60:305

Klingmüller D, Menger D, Wildt L, Leyendecker G, Krück F, Schweikert HU (1983) Induction of puberty in patients with Kallmann's syndrome. In: Leyendecker G, Stock H, Wildt L (eds) Brain and pituitary peptides II. Second Ferring symposium on brain and pituitary peptides, Kiel 1982. Karger, Basel, p 156

Klingmüller D, Schweikert HU (1985) Maintenance of spermatogenesis by intranasal administration of gonadotropin-releasing hormone in patients with hypothalamic hypogonadism. J Clin Endocrinol Metab 61:868

Krey LC, Butler WR, Knobil E (1975) Surgical disconnection of the medial basal hypothalamus and pituitary function in the rhesus monkey. I. Gonadotropin secretion. Endocrinology 96:1073

Leyendecker G, Wildt L, Hansmann M (1980) Pregnancies following chronic intermittent (pulsatile) administration of Gn-RH by means of a portable pump. („Zyklomat")−a new approach to the treatment of infertility in hypothalamic amenorrhea. J Clin Endocrinol Metab 51:1214

Miyachi Y, Mecklenburg RS, Hansen JW, Lipsett MB (1973) Metabolism of ^{125}I-luteinizing hormone-releasing hormone. J Clin Endocrinol Metab 37:63

Nikolics K, Mason AJ, Szoniy E, Ramachandran J, Seeburg PH (1985) A prolactin-inhibiting factor within the precursor for human gonadotropin-releasing hormone. Nature 316:511

Pimstone B, Epstein S, Hamilton SM, LeRoith D, Hendricks S (1977) Metabolic clearance and plasma half disappearance time of exogenous gonadotropin releasing hormone in normal subjects and in patients with liver disease and chronic renal failure. J Clin Endocrinol Metab 44:356

Santen RJ, Bardin CW (1973) Episodic luteinizing hormone secretin in man. Pulse analysis, clinical interpretation, physiological mechanisms. J Clin Invest 52:2617

Schrey MP (1985) Gonadotropin releasing hormone stimulates the formation of inositol phosphates in rat anterior pituitary tissue. Biochem J 226:563

Smith MA, Vale WW (1981) Desensitization to gonadotropin-releasing hormone observed in superfused pituitary cells on cytodex beads. Endocrinology 108:752

Wilson RC, Kesner JS, Kaufman J-M, Uemura T, Akema T, Knobil E (1983) Central electrophysiologic correlates of pulsatile luteinizing hormone secretion in the rhesus monkey. Neuroendocrinology 39:256

Direct Antitumor Effects of LH-RH Analogs

J. A. Foekens and J. G. M. Klijn

Division of Endocrine Oncology (Department of Medical Oncology),
Dr. Daniel den Hoed Cancer Center, P.O. Box 5201, 3008 AE Rotterdam, The Netherlands

Introduction

Luteinizing hormone releasing hormone (LH-RH) is a hypothalamic decapeptide secreted in a pulsatile way which leads to an increase in pituitary LH-RH receptor numbers and gonadotropin secretion [1]. Exposure of the pituitary gland to supraphysiological concentrations of LH-RH or continuously to long-acting LH-RH agonists causes downregulation of LH-RH receptors and loss of responsiveness (see review [2]). The presence of LH-RH or LH-RH-like peptides has not only been detected in the hypothalamus, but also in human biological fluids, the central nervous system, and a variety of normal and tumor tissues (see review [3]). This, together with the presence of LH-RH receptors in a wide range of normal and tumor tissues [3], has resulted in the suggestion that LH-RH may have a paracrine or autocrine role in the local regulation of cell biological processes. In the present report we summarize the literature with special emphasis on direct antitumor actions of LH-RH analogs on classical hormone-regulated cancers, i.e., of the breast, the prostate, and the ovaries.

Breast Cancer

Premenopausal breast cancer patients have successfully been treated with LH-RH analogs [4], and a large body of literature is currently available [2, 5, 6]. It is likely that beneficial clinical effects are achieved by suppressing the pituitary-ovarian axis [7] since this treatment reduces circulating estrogen to castrate levels [4]. Therefore, major clinical studies have been performed in premenopausal patients. However, LH-RH agonist treatment has also been successful in a minority of postmenopausal patients with advanced breast cancer, suggesting it has direct antitumor effects, but conflicting results have also been obtained [5, 8–13]. The existence of direct antitumor effects of LH-RH analogs is supported by the following findings: (a) the presence of LH-RH or

Recent Results in Cancer Research, Vol. 124
© Springer-Verlag Berlin · Heidelberg 1992

its activity in human milk and mammary tumor cells, (b) the presence of specific LH-RH binding sites in human mammary tumor cells and primary breast tumors, and (c) its direct biological effects in vitro.

LH-RH has been detected in human milk [14, 15] at levels 5- to 6-fold higher that in plasma as measured with a double antibody radioimmunoassay [14]. LH-RH-like immunoreactivity was identified in 7 of 11 human ductal adenocarcinomas of the mammary gland studied [16], and LH-RH and its messenger RNA (mRNA) were also detected in some human breast cancer cell lines [17, 18]. More recently, LH-RH immunoreactivity was found in 14 of 39 (36%) human breast tumor biopsies [19]. The immunostaining was found to be associated with the cytoplasm, the nucleus, or with both cell compartments. It was found in tumors of different histologic types. Interestingly, somatostatin, adrenocorticotropin-releasing hormone (CRH), and growth hormone releasing hormone (GH-RH) immunoreactivity was also present in 27%–35% of breast tumor biopsies [19]. Unlike these last three peptides, LH-RH immunoreactivity was found more frequently in breast tumors positive for estrogen and progesterone receptors. Of ten samples of atypical hyperplasia, somatostatin reactivity was detectable in four, of CRH in two, GH-RH in one, and LH-RH in none. All four peptides were absent in seven normal tissue samples analyzed [19].

Specific LH-RH binding sites have been demonstrated in human breast cancer cells in vitro and in human breast tumor biopsies [20–26]. Miller and associates [20, 22], using whole cell preparations of MCF-7 cells and the ^{125}I-labeled LH-RH agonist buserelin, detected specific low-affinity binding sites (K_d 10^{-4}–10^{-5} M). Two LH-RH antagonists competed for binding of labeled agonist with an approximately 10-fold higher affinity [20, 22]. Various other human breast cancer cell lines with different steroid receptor phenotypes in vitro (T-47D, MDA-MB-231, ZR75.1, Sk Br 3, MDA-MB-157) have subsequently been shown to contain LH-RH binding sites with moderately to low affinity [22, 23, 26]. In human breast carcinomas, and using another LH-RH agonist, specific binding sites (K_d $\approx 10^{-8}$ M) with a molecular weight of 64 000 were found to be present in 67% of the samples, as established by means of a ligand immunoblotting technique [21]. The incidence was higher in ductal carcinoma (86%) than in lobular carcinoma (22%). These LH-RH binding sites were not detectable in normal breast tissue [21]. Using multiple-point Scatchard analysis, 52% of breast tumor biopsies analyzed were classified as positive for LH-RH receptors [24]. No relationships were found between LH-RH receptor and epidermal growth factor (EGF) receptor, somatostatin receptor, or steroid receptors [24]. The potent agonist [D-Trp^6]-LH-RH bound to at least two classes of receptor site, one with low affinity and one with high affinity, both in rat pituitary and in human breast cancer samples [25]. Several unlabeled LH-RH antagonists were at least as effective as the potent agonist [D-Trp^6]-LH-RH in competing with [^{125}I-D-Trp^6]-LH-RH for binding to both classes of binding site in rat pituitary and human breast tumor membrane preparations. Using ^{125}I-LH-RH as the ligand, only one binding site with low to moderate affinity (K_d ≈ 50 μM) was detected in human breast cancer membranes. Labeled antagonists showed somewhat less affinity to membranes of pituitaries and breast cancers than the agonists and bound to only a single class of receptor sites [25].

Direct biological effects of LH-RH agonists and antagonists on breast cancer cells in vitro have been demonstrated [20, 22, 23, 26–36]. Initially, direct growth-inhibitory effects of LH-RH agonists were demonstrated for mouse mammary tumor cells in vitro [27, 28]. We have demonstrated that estradiol-stimulated growth of MCF-7 human breast cancer cells could be inhibited by the LH-RH agonist buserelin in a dose-dependent manner [29–31, 33–35]. Wiznitzer and Benz [32], in a preliminary study, reported growth-inhibitory effects of an LH-RH agonist with respect to prolactin-stimulated proliferation of T-47D breast cancer cells. Miller and coworkers [20, 22] not only found inhibition of MCF-7 cell proliferation but even a net decrease in cell number at buserelin concentrations ranging from 1 nM to 1 µM. In contrast, concentrations of buserelin which were inhibitory in MCF-7 cells were totally ineffective against MDA-MB-231 cells and produced minimal effects in the T-47D cell cultures [22]. In MCF-7 cells we found no effect of buserelin on the levels of cytoplasmic and nuclear estrogen receptors, on the pattern of [^{35}S]methionine labeled secretory proteins, or on the secretion of proteins with EGF-like activities [33–35], whereas the level of estrogen-induced progesterone receptor was decreased [33, 34]. The inhibitory effect of buserelin on the estradiol-stimulated growth of MCF-7 cells could partly be abolished by the antiestrogen tamoxifen [33]. Both Miller et al. [20, 22] and our group [30, 33, 34] have shown that concomitant administration of LH-RH antagonists prevented the growth-inhibitory effects of the LH-RH agonist. However, Eidne and coworkers [23] observed no effects on [^{3}H]thymidine uptake into ZR75.1 cells of various LH-RH agonists, while other LH-RH antagonists were able to cause an approximately 40% inhibition of [^{3}H]thymidine incorporation. These studies of Eidne and associates have recently been substantiated by Sharoni et al. [36], who also showed that two LH-RH antagonists caused inhibition of [^{3}H]thymidine incorporation by up to 40% in MDA-MB-231 cells after 2 days of incubation, whereas buserelin was not effective in this respect. In contrast, another LH-RH agonist (ovulerin) has recently been shown to be effective on the proliferation of MDA-MB-231 cells in vitro [26]. Moreover, immunosuppressed mice bearing either MCF-7 or MDA-MB-231 xenografts responded to high-doses of the LH-RH agonist zoladex depot and to decapeptyl depot therapy [26]. Similarly, in vivo, an LH-RH agonist caused a decrease in the labeling index from 12 to 48 h after administration in ovariectomized hypophysectomized mice with MXT mammary tumors [37]. On the other hand, with MCF-7 cells cultured in vitro in serum-free medium, we found no effect of LH-RH agonist on the amount of S-phase cells after 48 h, both in cultures lacking estradiol and in the presence of estradiol. In studies with ovariectomized immature rats, no antiestrogenic effects of LH-RH agonists were found [38], and also no tumor growth-inhibiting effects of intratumoral LH-RH implants in dimethylbenzanthracene-(DMBA)-induced rat mammary tumors were observed [39]. In contrast, other investigators did report a direct effect of LH-RH analogs on estrogen-responsive DMBA-induced mammary tumors in the rat [40].

In summary, with breast tumor cells, both in vitro and in vivo, conflicting reports have appeared in the literature with respect to direct growth-inhibitory effects of LH-RH analogs. The majority of the studies are in favor of the existence of such a direct effect on various breast tumor cells. The discrepancies in the in vitro studies may partly be explained by the variation in clonal cell lines used in the various laboratories [41]. Moreover, different culture conditions used by various investigators may underlie the discrepancies. For instance, in our own experience, larger stimulatory effects of estradiol and more potent inhibition of these stimulated cultures by buserelin were observed [33, 34] in experiments using human serum than in experiments with fetal calf serum as a medium supplement [30]. Moreover, it has been reported that insulin, normally used as an additive in the in vitro culture of human breast cancer cells, could overrule the inhibitory effects caused by the LH-RH agonist [22]. It is attractive to assume that the tumor remissions observed in some postmenopausal breast cancer patients as a response to LH-RH agonist treatment are due to a direct tumor growth inhibitory effect. However, the observed decrease in plasma testosterone [13, 42], a substrate for peripheral synthesis of estradiol, may have caused the objective tumor remissions in postmenopausal patients observed in some of the studies.

Prostate Cancer

Various clinical trials have documented that buserelin, goserelin, [D-Trp[6]]-LH-RH and leuprolide can be successfully used for palliative treatment of patients with advanced prostate carcinoma (see reviews [43, 44]). As in the treatment of premenopausal breast cancer patients, the effects are caused by blockade of the pituitary-gonadal axis. Regarding direct tumor growth inhibitory effects of LH-RH analogs, we have reported that androgen-stimulated growth of LNCaP human prostate cancer cells in vitro was inhibited by 0.8 μM buserelin [34]. This inhibitory effect of buserelin on cell proliferation was observed when the cells were stimulted with low concentrations of androgen ($10^{-11}\ M$ R1881), but not in the presence of a 10-fold higher concentration [34]. Schally and Redding, using the same cell line, also observed inhibition of cell proliferation caused by $10^{-2}-10^{-6}\ M$ tryptorelin [45]. The same group of investigators showed inhibition of [^{3}H]thymidine uptake caused by $10^{-5}-10^{-7}\ M$ concentrations of the LH-RH agonist [D-Trp[6]]-LH-RH in two other prostate tumor cell lines (DU-145, PC-3) [45, 46]. In addition, using [^{125}I-D-Trp[6]]-LH-RH, they demonstrated the presence of specific receptors for LH-RH in the Dunning rat prostate tumor [47-49], human prostate tumors [48-50], and in 1 out of 13 benign prostatic hypertrophy (BPH) samples [49]. LH-RH receptors were not detected in eight specimens of normal human prostate [49]. Both in the Dunning prostate tumor and in the human prostate tumors, two classes of binding sites were present, one with a high affinity ($K_d \approx 10^{-10}\ M$) and one with a moderately to low affinity (K_d 10^{-6} to 8×10^{-8} M) for [^{125}I-D-Trp^6]-LH-RH [49]. Interestingly, treatment of rats carrying the prostate Dunning R-3327 tumor with microcapsules of [D-Trp^6]-LH-RH increased the binding capacity of the low-affinity binding sites and in addition decreased the levels of measurable high-affinity [D-Trp^6]-LH-RH binding sites [49]. These data are similar to those obtained in in vitro studies by Scaletzky et al. [51], who showed that low-affinity LH-RH receptors (K_d 10^{-6} M) of LNCaP human prostate tumor cells were increased in a dose-dependent manner upon incubation of the cells with an LH-RH agonist. Recently, LH-RH-like activity has also been demonstrated in conditioned media from an androgen-insensitive (DU145) and from an androgen-responsive (LNCaP) human prostate cancer cell line [52]. In addition, the same study also reported the presence of LH-RH-like activity in concentrated cytosols of human prostatic tumor and BPH biopsies. Although the mean content was significantly higher in cytosols from malignant tissues ($\approx$3-fold higher) when compared to benign tissues, more specimens of benign tissues (37 of 54 positive) than of malignant tissue (6 of 22) were positive for LH-RH-like activity [52].

In summary, the presence of LH-RH receptors and LH-RH-like activities in prostatic tumor tissues and the absence of LH-RH receptors (and LH-RH-like activity?) in normal prostatic tissues may suggest that LH-RH acts as a growth factor and may be involved in the promotion of prostate cancer in man. The observed direct growth inhibitory effects of LH-RH agonists on the proliferation of human prostate cancer cells suggests that part of the beneficial clinical effect observed in the treatment of advanced prostate cancer may have been due to direct antitumor effects. Therefore, for the minority of cases of prostate cancer which are negative for androgen receptors, chronic LH-RH administration may cause objective remissions, in analogy with the treatment of postmenopausal breast cancer patients.

Ovarian Cancer

In 1982, Lamberts et al. [53] described a direct inhibitory effect of an LH-RH agonist (ICI 118630) on steroidogenesis in cultured primary arrhenoblastoma cells. This inhibiting effect of an LH-RH agonist suggested that LH-RH receptors were present on these tumor cells, and the authors discussed whether treatment with LH-RH agonists might be beneficial in patients with metastatic steroid hormone-secreting ovarian and testicular tumors [53]. Thus, the observed direct antitumor effects of LH-RH agonists on the proliferation of human breast cancer cells in particular (as discussed above), and the observation that the proliferation of ovarian cancer cells in vitro was stimulated by human chorionic gonadotropin (hCG) and follicle-stimulating hormone (FSH) [54, 55], have produced a greater interest in the use of LH-RH agonists in ovarian cancer. Several clinical studies performed subsequently with LH-RH agonists have demonstrated some beneficial effect in the treatment of advanced ovarian cancer (see reviews [56, 57]). Kullander et al. [58] and Pour et al. [59] reported inhibition of growth of experimental animal tumors using the LH-RH agonist [D-Trp^6]-LH-RH. The growth of the human ovarian cancer cell line OVCAR-3 in nude mice was also inhibited after administration of [D-Trp^6]-LH-RH [60]. An LH-RH-like protein distinct from LH-RH has been described in luteinized rat ovaries [61]. High-affinity receptors for LH-RH have shown to be present on rat ovarian cell membranes and direct antigonadotropic effects on cultured rat granulosa and luteal cells have been described [62–65]. The presence of an LH-RH-like protein in extracts of human ovaries [66] as well as the presence of LH-RH binding sites associated with human corpus luteum [67, 68] have been reported. Only in recent years has the presence of specific LH-RH binding sites been reported for human ovarian carcinoma tissues [56, 69–71]. In photoaffinity labeling experiments, Pahwa et al. [69] showed specific binding of the LH-RH agonist [D-Lys^6]-LH-RH to be associated with a high molecular weight protein of 63 000. A single class of specific LH-RH agonist binding sites with a low affinity ($K_d \approx 7 \times 10^{-6}$ M) could be demonstrated in plasma membranes from 32 of 40 (80%) ovarian carcinoma samples tested [70]. With respect to direct growth-inhibitory effects of LH-RH agonists on ovarian cancer cells in vitro, no positive but one negative report showing negligible direct antitumor effects is thus far available in the literature [72]. The proliferation of isolated normal human ovarian cells grown in vitro were not or only marginally affected by LH-RH [73, 74].

In summary, it is at present unclear whether the tumor growth inhibition observed in patients with advanced ovarian cancer was caused by a direct effect or by indirect endocrine effects due to lowering of plasma LH and FSH, or by a combination of these effects. Suppression of the secretion of gonadotropins induced by LH-RH agonists has been shown to inhibit the growth of epithelial ovarian cancers [43, 71]. It is promising that chronic treatment with [D-Trp^6]-LH-RH microcapsules induced the regression of an inoperable, bilateral, serous cystadenocarcinoma of the ovary in a 78-year-old woman [75], and moreover caused a remission or stabilization of disease in 11 of 39 patients with epithelial ovarian cancer [76]. Schally and Redding [45] discussed whether LH-RH agonist treatment may also be useful for treating patients with advanced ovarian cancer who have relapsed after chemotherapy and for those who cannot tolerate chemotherapy.

Conclusions

Specific binding sites for LH-RH (agonists) are present in human breast, prostate, ovarian, and endometrial cancer [77] tissues. Most of these tumor types, or their normal counterparts, also contain LH-RH-like activities. It is, therefore, possible that LH-RH may act as an paracrine or autocrine (transforming?) growth factor in these cancers. The low-affinity character of the receptor in human tumor tissues, as measured in most of the studies, has prompted several authors to suggest that these receptors can only be of minor importance regarding the peripheral concentrations of LH-RH analogs which would be needed to induce an effect. One should, however, keep in mind that receptor binding studies were performed either on whole cell preparations of cells cultured in vitro or on isolated tissue membrane preparations. Obviously this non-in situ situation could have affected the binding behavior of the ligand to such a large molecule as the receptor, particularly with respect to its affinity. The direct inhibitory effects of LH-RH analogs on the proliferation of some types of cancer cells in vitro are important from a biological point of view, but – with a few exceptions – are probably of low significance in the palliative treatment of humans with advanced disease. By contrast, the presence of LH-RH receptors may indeed have important clinical applications, i.e., it may enable localization of tumors or metastases with tracer amounts of radioactive agonists, as has been shown for a variety of somatostatin-receptor-positive tumors with radioactive somatostatin analogs by scanning techniques [78, 79].

References

1. Clayton RN (1982) Gonadotropin-releasing hormone modulation of its own pituitary receptors: evidence for biphasic regulation. Endocrinology 111:152
2. Furr BJA, Woodburn JR (1988) Luteinizing hormone-releasing hormone an its analogues: a review of biological properties and clinical uses. J Endocrinol Invest 11:535
3. Klijn JGM, Foekens JA (1989) Extrapituitary actions. In: Vickery BH, Lunenfeld B (eds) GnRH analogues in cancer and human reproduction, vol 1, Basic aspects. Kluwer, Dordrecht, p 71
4. Klijn JGM, de Jong FH (1982) Treatment with a luteinizing-hormone-releasing-hormone analogue (buserelin) in premenopausal patients with metastatic breast cancer. Lancet i:1213
5. Manni A, Santen R, Harvey H, Lipton A, Max D (1986) Treatment of breast cancer with gonadotropin-releasing hormone. Endocr Rev 7:89
6. Klijn JGM, Foekens JA (1988) Long-term peptide hormone treatment with LH-RH agonists in metastatic breast cancer. In: Santen RJ, Juhos E (eds) Endocrine-dependent breast cancer: critical assessment of recent advances. Huber, Toronto, p 92
7. Schally AV, Arimura A, Coy AH (1980) Recent approaches to fertility control based on derivatives of LH-RH. Vitam Horm 38:257
8. Harvey HA, Lipton A, Max DT (1984) LH-RH analogs for human mammary carcinoma. In: Vickery BH, Nestor JJ, Hafez ESE (eds) LH-RH and its analogs, contraceptive and clinical application. MTP, Lancaster, p 329
9. Schwartz L, Guiochet N, Keiling R (1988) Two partial remissions induced by an LHRH analogue in two postmenopausal women with metastatic breast cancer. Cancer 62:2498
10. Plowman PN, Nicholson RI, Walker KJ (1986) Remissions of metastatic breast cancer in postmenopausal women with luteinizing hormone releasing hormone (ICI 118630) therapy. Eur J Cancer Clin Oncol 22:746
11. Waxman JH, Harlend SJ, Coombes RC, Wrigley PFM, Malpas JS, Powles T, Lister TA (1985) The treatment of postmenopausal women with advanced breast cancer with buserelin. Cancer Chemother Pharmacol 15:171
12. Harris AL, Carmichael J, Cantwell, Dowsett M (1989) Zoladex: endocrine and therapeutic effects in post-menopausal breast cancer. Br J Cancer 59:97
13. Crighton IL, Dowsett M, Lai A, Man A, Smith IE (1989) Use of luteinising hormone-releasing hormone agonist (leuprolin) in advanced post-menopausal breast cancer: clinical and endocrine effects. Br J Cancer 60:644
14. Sarda AK, Nair RMG (1981) Elevated levels of LRH in human milk. J Clin Endocrinol Metab 52:647

14   J. A. Foekens and J. G. M. Klijn

15. Amarant T, Fridkin M, Koch Y (1982) Luteinizing hormone-releasing hormone and thyrotropin releasing hormone in human and bovine milk. Eur J Biochem 127:647
16. Seppälä M, Wahlström T (1980) Identification of luteinizing hormone-releasing factor and alpha subunit of glycoprotein hormones in ductal carcinoma of the mammary gland. Int J Cancer 26:267
17. Bützow R, Huhtaniemi I, Clayton R, Wahlström T, Andersson LC, Seppälä M (1987) Cultured mammary carcinoma cells contain gonadotropin-releasing hormone-like immunoreactivity, GnRH binding sites and chorionic gonadotropin. Int J Cancer 39:498
18. Eidne KA, Harris NS, Millar RP, Wilcox J (1987) GnRH-immunoreactivity and GnRH m-RNA in two human breast cancer cell lines MDA-MB-231 and ZR-75-1. 69th Annual Meeting of the Endocrine Society, Indianapolis, 10–12 June, 653
19. Ciocca DR, Puy La, Fasoli LC, Tello O, Aznar JC, Gago FE, Papa SI, Soneho R (1990) Corticotropin-releasing hormone, luteinizing hormone-releasing hormone, and somatostatin-like immunoreactivities in biopsies from breast cancer patients. Breast Cancer Res Treat 15:175
20. Miller WR, Scott WN, Morris R, Fraser HM, Sharpe RM (1985) Growth of human breast cancer cells inhibited by a luteinizing hormone-releasing hormone agonist. Nature 313:231
21. Eidne KA, Flanagan CA, Millar RP (1985) Gonadotropin-releasing hormone binding sites in human breast carcinoma. Science 229:989
22. Miller WR, Scott WN, Fraser HM, Sharpe RM (1987) Direct inhibition of human breast cancer cell growth by an LHRH agonist. In: Klijn JGM, Paridaens R, Foekens JA (eds) Hormonal manipulation of cancer: peptides, growth factors, and new (anti) steroidal agents. Raven, New York, p 357 (EORTC monograph series, vol 18)
23. Eidne KA, Flanagan CA, Harris NS, Millar RP (1987) Gonadotropin-releasing hormone (GnRH)-binding sites in human breast cancer cell lines and inhibitory effects of GnRH antagonists. J Clin Endocrinol Metab 64:425
24. Fekete M, Wittliff JL, Schally AV (1989) Characterization and distribution of receptors for [D-Trp[6]]-luteinizing-hormone-releasing hormone, somatostatin, epidermal growth factor, and sex steroids in 500 biopsy samples of human breast cancer. J Clin Lab Analysis 3:137
25. Fekete M, Bajusz S, Groot K, Csernus VJ, Schally AV (1989) Comparison of different agonists and antagonists of luteinizing hormone-releasing hormone for receptor-binding ability to rat pituitary and human breast cancer membranes. Endocrinoloty 124:946
26. Vincze B, Pályi I, Daubner D, Kremmer T, Számel I, Bodrogi I, Sugár J, Seprôdi J, Mezô I, Teplán I, Eckhardt S (1991) Influence of luteinizing hormone-releasing hormone agonists on human mammary carcinoma cell lines and their xenografts. J Steroid Biochem Mol Biol 38:119
27. Corbin A (1982) From contraception to cancer: a review of the therapeutic applications of LH-RH analogues as antitumor agents. Yale J Biol Med 55:27
28. Matsuzawa A, Yamamoto T (1982) Enhanced and reversed growth in vitro of a pregnancy-dependent mouse mammary tumor (TPDMT-4) by a gonadotropin-releasing hormone agonist analog. Eur J Cancer Clin Oncol 18:495
29. Blankenstein MA, Henkelman MS, Klijn JGM (1983) An analogue of LHRH antagonizes the growth-stimulatory effect of estradiol on human breast cancer cells in culture (MCF-7). J Steroid Biochem 19 (Suppl):95 S
30. Blankenstein MA, Henkelman MS, Klijn JGM (1985) Direct inhibitory effect of a luteinizing hormone-releasing hormone agonist on MCF-7 human breast cancer cells. Eur J Cancer Clin Oncol 21:1493
31. Klijn JGM, de Jong FH, Lamberts SWJ, Blankenstein MA (1985) LHRH-agonist treatment in clinical and experimental human breast cancer. J Steroid Biochem 23:867
32. Wiznitzer I, Benz L (1984) Direct growth inhibiting effects of the prolactin antagonist buserelin and pergolide on human breast cancer. Proc Am Assoc Cancer Res 25:208
33. Foekens JA, Henkelman MS, Fukkink JF, Blankenstein MA, Klijn JGM (1986) Combined effects of buserelin, estradiol and tamoxifen on the growth of MCF-7 human breast cancer cells in vitro. Biochem Biophys Res Commun 140:550

34. Foekens JA, Henkelman MS, Bolt-de Vries J, Portengen H, Fukkink JF, Blankenstein MA, van Steenbrugge GJ, Mulder E, Klijn JGM (1987) Direct effects of LHRH analogs on breast and prostate tumor cells. In: Klijn JGM, Paridaens R, Foekens JA (eds) Hormonal manipulation of cancer: peptides, growth factors, and new (anti) steroidal agents. Raven, New York, p 369 (EORTC monograph series, vol 18)

35. Foekens JA, Klijn JGM (1988) Direct antitumor effects of an LH-RH agonist. In: Höffken K (ed) LH-RH agonists in oncology. Springer, Berlin Heidelberg New York, p 22

36. Sharoni Y, Bosin E, Miinster A, Levy J, Schally AV (1989) Inhibition of growth of human mammary tumor cells by potent antagonists of luteinizing hormone-releasing hormone. Proc Natl Acad Sci USA 86:1648

37. De Launoit Y, Kiss R, Danguy A, Paridaens R (1987) Effects of ovariectomy, hypophysectomy and/or GnRH analog (HRF) administration on the cell proliferation of the MXT mouse hormone-dependent mammary tumor. Eur J Cancer Clin Oncol 23:1443

38. Furr BJA, Nicholson RI (1982) Use of analogs of luteinizing hormone-releasing hormone for the treatment of cancer. J Reprod Fert 64:529

39. Nicholson RI, Walker KJ, Turkes A, Dyas J, Gotting KE, Plowman PM, Williams M, Elston CW, Blamey RW (1987). The British experience with the LH-RH agonist Zoladex (ICI 118630) in the treatment of breast cancer. In: Klijn JGM, Paridaens R, Foekens JA (eds) Hormonal manipulation of cancer: peptides, growth factors, and new (anti) steroidal agents. Raven, New York, p 331 (EORTC Monograph Series, vol 18)

40. Segal T, Levy J, Sharoni Y (1987) GnRH analogs stimulate phospholipase C activity in mammary tumor membranes: modulation by GTP. Mol Cell Endocrinol 53:239

41. Wilding G, Chen M, Gelman EP (1987) LHRH agonists and human breast cancer cells. Nature 329:770

42. Dowsett M, Cantwell B, Lal A, Jeffcoate SL, Harris AL (1988) Suppression of postmenopausal ovarian steroidogenesis with the luteinizing hormone-releasing hormone agonist goserelin. J Clin Endocrinol Metab 66:672

43. Schally AV, Bajusz S, Redding TW, Zalatnai A, Comaru-Schally AM (1989) Analogs of LHRH: the present and the future. In: Vickery BH, Lunenfeld V (eds) GnRH analogues in cancer and human reproduction, vol 1, Basic aspects. Kluwer, Dordrecht, p 5

44. Schally AV, Srkalovic G, Szende B, Redding TW, Janaky T, Juhasz A, Korkut E, Cai RZ, Szepeshazi K, Radulovic S, Bokser L, Groot K, Serfozo P, Comaru-Schally AM (1990) Antitumor effects of anlogs of LH-RH and somatostatin: experimental and clinical studies. J Steoid Biochem Mol Biol 37:1061

45. Schally AV, Redding TW (1987) Use of LH-RH analogs for the treatment of prostate cancer: combination therapy and direct effects. In: Klijn JGM, Paridaens R, Foekens JA (eds) Hormonal manipulation of cancer: peptides, growth factors, and new (anti) steroidal agents. Raven, New York, p 273 (EORTC Monograph Series, vol 18)

46. Schally AV, Redding TW, Paz-Bouza JI, Comaru-Schally AM, Mathé G (1987) Current consept for improving treatment of prostate cancer based on combination of LH-RH agonists with other agents. In: Murphy G, Küss R, Khoury S, Chatelain C, Denis L (eds) Prostate cancer part A: research endocrine treatment and histopathology. Liss, New York, p 173

47. Hierowski MT, Altamirano P. Redding TW, Schally AV (1983) The presence of LHRH-like receptors in Dunning R3327H prostate tumors. FEBS Lett 154:92

48. Kadar T, Redding TW, Ben-David M, Schally AV (1988) Receptors for prolactin, somatostatin, and luteinizing hormone-releasing hormone in experimental prostate cancer after treatment with analogs of luteinizing hormone-releasing hormone and somatostatin. Proc Natl Acad Sci USA 85:890

49. Fekete M, Redding TW, Comaru-Schally AM, Pontes JE, Connelly RW, Srkalovic G, Schally AV (1989) Receptors for luteinizing hormone-releasing hormone, somatostatin, prolactin, and epidermal growth factor in rat and human prostate cancers and in benign prostate hyperplasia. Prostate 14:191

50. Kadar T, Ben-Davin M, Pontes JE, Fekete M, Dchally AV (1968) Prolactin and luteinizing hormone-releasing hormone receptors in human benign prostatic hyperplasia and prostate cancer. Prostate 12:299

51. Scaletzky R, Qayum A, Clayton RN, Sikora K, Waxman J (1988) GnRH analogue and dihydrotestosterone treatment regulate expression of GnRH binding in a human hormone dependent prostatic cancer cell line. Gynecol Endocrinol 2 (Suppl 1):100
52. Quayum A, Gullick WJ, Mellon K, Krausz T, Neal D, Sikora K, Waxman J (1990) The partial purification and characterization of GnRH-like activity from prostatic biopsy specimens and prostatic cancer cell lines. J Steroid Biochem Mol Biol 37:899
53. Lamberts SWJ, Timmers JM, Oosterom R, Verleun T, Rommerts FG, de Jong FH (1982) Testosterone secretion by cultured arrhenoblastoma cells: suppression by a luteinizing hormone-releasing hormone agonist. J Clin Endocrinol Metab 54:450
54. Simon WE, Hölzel F (1979) Hormone sensitivity of gynecological tumor cells in tissue cultures. J Cancer Res Clin Oncol 94:307
55. Simon WE, Albrecht M, Hänzel M, Dietel M, Hölzel F (1983) Cell lines derived from human ovarian carcinomas: growth stimulation by gonadotropic hormones. J Natl Cancer Inst 70:839
56. Emons G, Pahwa GS, Ortmann O, Knuppen R, Oberheuser F, Schultz K-D (1990) LHRH-receptors and LHRH-agonist treatment in ovarian cancer. J Steroid Biochem Mol Biol 37:1003
57. Rao BR, Slotman BJ (1991) Endocrine factors in common epithelial ovarian cancer. Endocr Rev 12:14
58. Kullander S, Rausing A, Schally AV (1987) LHRH agonist treatment in ovarian cancer. In: Klijn JGM, Paridaens R, Foekens JA (eds) Hormonal manipulation of cancer: peptides, growth factors, and new (anti) steroidal agents. Raven, New York, p 353 (EORTC monograph series, vol 18)
59. Pour PM, Redding TW, Paz-Bouza JI, Schally AV (1988) Treatment of experimental ovarian carcinoma with monthly injection of the agonist D-Trp⁶-LH-RH: a preliminary report. Cancer Lett 41:105
60. Mortel R, Satyaswaroop PG, Schally AV, Hamilton T, Ozols R (1986) Inhibitory effects of GnRH superagonist on the growth of human ovarian carcinoma NIH: OVCAR-3 in the nude mouse. Gynaecol Oncol 23:254
61. Aten RF, Williams AT, Behrman HR (1986) Ovarian gonadotropin-releasing hormone-like protein(s): demonstration and characterization. Endocrinology 118:961
62. Behrman HR, Preston SL, Hall AK (1980) Cellular mechanism of the antigonadotropic action of luteinizing hormone-releasing hormone in the corpus luteum. Endocrinology 107:656
63. Jones PBC, Conn PM, Marian J, Hsueh AJW (1980) Binding of gonadotropin releasing hormone agonist to rat ovarian granulosa cell cells. Life Sci 27:2125
64. Clayton RN, Harwood JP, Catt KJ (1979) Gonadotropin-releasing hormone analogue binds to luteal cells and inhibits progesterone production. Nature 282:90
65. Hsueh AJW, Jones PBC (1981) Extrapituitary actions of gonadotropin-releasing hormone. Endocr Rev 2:437
66. Aten RF, Polan ML, Bayless R, Behrman HR (1987) A gonadotropin-releasing hormone (GnRH)-like protein in human ovaries: similarity to the GnRH-like ovarian protein of the rat. J Clin Endocrinol Metab 64:1288
67. Popkin R, Bramley TA, Currie A, Shaw RW, Baird DT, Frazer (1983). Specific binding of luteinizing hormone releasing hormone to human luteal tissue. Biochem Biophys Res Commun 114:750
68. Bramley TA, Menzies GS, Baird DT (1985) Specific binding of gonadotropin-releasing hormone and an agonist to human corpus luteum homogenates: characterization, properties, and luteal phase levels. J Clin Endocrinol Metab 61:834
69. Pahwa GS, Vollmer G, Knuppen R, Emons G (1989) Photoaffinity labelling of gonadotropin releasing hormone binding sites in human epithelial ovarian carcinomata. Biochem Biophys Res Commun 161:1086
70. Emons G, Pahwa GS, Brack C, Sturm R, Oberhauser F, Knuppen R (1989) Gonadotropin releasing hormone binding sites in human epithelial ovarian carcinomata. Eur J Cancer Clin Oncol 25:215

71. Parmar H, Phillips RH, Rustin G, Lightman SL, Schally AV (1988) Therapy of advanced ovarian cancer with D-Trp-6-LHRH (decapeptyl) microcapsules. Biomed Pharmacother 42:531
72. Slotman BJ, Poels LG, Rao BR (1989) A direct LHRH-agonist action on cancer cells is unlikely to be the case of response to LHRH-agonist therapy. Anticancer Res 9:77
73. Hsueh AJW, Schaeffer JM (1985) Gonadotropin-releasing hormone as a paracrine hormone and neurotransmitter in extra-pituitary sites. J Steroid Biochem 23:757
74. Knecht M, Ranta T, Feng P, Shinohara O, Catt KJ (1985) Gonadotropin-releasing hormone as a modulator of ovarian function. J Steroid Biochem 23:771
75. Parmar H, Nicoll J, Stockdale A, Cassoni A, Phillips RH, Lightman SL, Schally AV (1985) Advanced ovarian carcinoma: response to the agonist D-Trp-6-LH-RH. Cancer Treat Rep 69:1341
76. Parmar H, Phillips RH, Rustin G, Hanham IW, Schally AV, Lightman SL (1988) Response to D-Trp-6-LHRH (decapeptyl) microcapsules in advanced ovarian cancer Br Med J 296:1229
77. Srkalovic G, Wittliff JL, Schally AV (1990) Detection and partial characterization of receptors for [D-Trp[6]]-luteinizing hormone-releasing hormone and epidermal growth factor in human endometrial carcinoma. Cancer Res 50:1841
78. Krenning EP, Bakker WH, Breeman WAP, Koper JW, Kooij PPM, Ausema L, Lameris JS, Reubi JC, Lamberts SWJ (1989) Localisation of endocrine-related tumours with radioiodinated analogue of somatostatin. Lancet i:242
79. Lamberts SWJ, Bakker WH, Reubi J-C, Krenning EP (1990) Somatostatin-receptor imaging in the localization of endocrine tumors. N Engl J Med 323:1246

LH-RH Agonists in Benign and Malignant Tumors

Treatment of Uterine Leiomyomata by LH-RH Agonists

Z. Blumenfeld

Reproductive Endocrinology & Infertility Section, Department of Obstetrics & Gynecology, Rambam Medical Center, Faculty of Medicine – Technion, Israel Institute of Technology, Haifa 31096, Israel

Introduction

The rapid development and availability of luteinizing hormone releasing hormone (LH-RH) agonists have led to their widespread utilization in a variety of gynecologic conditions (McLachlan et al. 1986). One of the most common conditions in the practice of the gynecologist is uterine leiomyomata (Heinrichs 1991). Uterine leiomyomata are the most common solid tumor of the female genital tract and may bring about menometrorrhagia, pelvic pain and discomfort, anemia, infertility and habitual abortion (Blumenfeld et al. 1990; Esterday et al. 1983; Filicori et al. 1983; Heinrichs 1991). Estrogens are known to play a major role in the development and enlargement of these tumors. High levels of estrogen receptors have been found in this type of tumor, and exogenous administration of estrogens may result in rapid increase in their size (Blumenfeld et al. 1990; Filicori et al. 1983; Heinrichs 1991; Tamaya et al. 1985; Wilson et al. 1980). The estrogen dependence is in agreement with the clinical observations that fibroids are most commonly diagnosed in women aged between 30 and 50 years, that fibroids tend to shrink after the menopause, and that fibroids can rapidly increase in size during pregnancy (Healy 1990). On the other hand, case-control analysis of 535 women who had had leiomyomata showed that the risk of leiomyomata was inversely correlated with the number of term pregnancies (Healy 1990; Ross et al. 1986). This suggested that low, unopposed estradiol (E_2) levels, resulting from the several pregnancies and also the subsequent puerperia, reduced the growth of nascent leiomyomata (Healy 1990). The risk of developing leiomyomata was directly correlated with increasing duration of oral contraceptive use, lower body weight, and cigarette smoking (Healy 1990; Ross et al. 1986). Serum E_2 concentrations in patients with uterine leiomyomata were similar to those in control women (Healy 1990; Soules and McCarthy 1982; Spellacy et al. 1972).

Uterine leiomyomata are present in 20%–25% of women 35 years of age and older, and are the major indication for hysterectomy (Heinrichs 1991). As with endometriosis, these benign tumors are estrogen dependent, occurring during the reproductive years and regressing after the menopause. Clinical symptoms of hypermenorrhea, e.g., pelvic pressure – perhaps provoking urinary frequency or obstruction to stool evacuation – backache, and perhaps relative infertility or pregnancy loss, are slowly progressive. During the fifth decade of life with its diminished corpus luteum function and increasing frequency of anovulatory cycles, the rate of growth of fibroids increases until estrogen levels fall during the perimenopause. Although the etiology of leiomyomata remains unknown, each tumor appears from cell culture data to be comprised of a single clone of cells. The concentration of E_2 receptors is greater in the tumors than in adjacent myometrium (Tamaya et al. 1985; Wilson et al. 1980).

Based on the hypothesis that hypoestrogenism induced by LH-RH agonists will result in regression of fibroid tumors, Filicori et al. (1983) reported a case in which a 77.5% reduction in size was observed. Healy et al. (1984) found in another instance that a subcutaneous infusion also dramatically reduced the volume of a leiomyomatous uterus. One year later, Maheux et al. (1985) announced a surprising 80% regression in 7 of 23 myomata identified among ten women treated daily with 500 µg buserelin subcutaneously for 6 months; two of the remaining tumors regressed by 25% and three remained unchanged in size. This pilot study was soon confirmed in six patients using daily subcutaneous injections of histerilin, which produced a 37%–65% reduction in size of leiomyomata in 6 months of therapy (Coddington et al. 1986; Healy 1990), and by intermittent subcutaneous infusion (Healy et al. 1986; Ross et al. 1986) of 400 µg buserelin three times daily intranasally, or by short-term treatment with microencapsulated [D-Trp⁶]-LH-RH (Van Leusden 1986). Shortly thereafter, a subcutaneous implant of goserelin (3.6 mg every 4 weeks) in 13 patients produced amenorrhea in two-thirds of them, and regression of myomata size averaged 55% (range, 38%–84%) (West et al. 1987). These results were achieved by suppressing E_2 to early follicular phase levels (mean value, 35 pg/ml), not to postmenopausal levels.

After the above pilot studies with three different analogs had been conducted, more than 20 reports of open-design, confirmatory studies appeared in the literature; more than 170 women participated (Blumenfeld et al. 1991; Heinrichs 1991). Most investigators used ultrasonography to document change in uterine and/or fibroid volume. Seven different analogs were utilized in a variety of doses, routes of administration, and durations, although most regimens lasted for 6 months. Reductions in uterine or fibroid volume ranged from a 50% decrease in size to complete absence (Heinrichs 1991; West et al. 1987). The consistent finding was a reduction of 40%–70% in tumor/uterine volume. Larger tumors shrank the most and more predictably than the smaller myomata (Andreyko et al. 1988; Donnez et al. 1989; Friedman et al. 1987; Friedman et al. 1989a, b; Friedman 1989b; George et al. 1989; Golan et al. 1989; Kessel et al. 1988; Letterie et al. 1989; Maheux et al. 1987, 1988; Perl et al. 1987; Van der Spuy et al. 1989; Vollenhoven et al. 1990; Williams and Shaw 1990). Monitoring uterine change by magnetic resonance imaging (Andreyko et al. 1988; Blumenfeld et al. 1990; Maheux et al. 1987; Williams and Shaw

1990), hysterography (Donnez et al. 1989), or ultrasonography (Blumenfeld et al. 1990; Williams and Shaw 1990) was confirmatory and offered additional information about intrinsic pathology or localization. Chronological evaluations indicated that the shrinkage that occurred was evident and nearly complete after 3 months of therapy; longer periods of therapy were not greatly beneficial (Blumenfeld et al. 1990; Friedman et al. 1988; Vollenhoven et al. 1990; Williams and Shaw 1990).

After cessation of therapy, most of the tumors grew to their previous size, or even larger, as ovulatory function was restored. Long-term observation of 19 treated perimenopausal women suggests that observation only may replace post-treatment hysterectomy for most women (Schlaff et al. 1989; Van Leusden 1988). A report by Friedman et al. (1989a, b) suggests that regrowth is prevented after 3 months of LH-RH agonist therapy by instituting a commonly used regimen of conjugated equine estrogens (0.625 mg orally daily for 25 days per month) and progestin (medroxyprogesterone acetate, 10 mg orally) during the last 10 days of the monthly estrogen. The tumors remained at end-of-treatment volume during 27 months of observation (Friedman 1989b). In contrast, medroxyprogesterone acetate given simultaneously as the LH-RH agonist throughout treatment prevented most of the initial reduction in size (15% – 18% versus 50% – 55%) (Friedman et al. 1988). This observation is in agreement with the similar response of endometriotic lesions when, in an attempt to reduce side effects, medroxyprogesterone acetate was introduced (Cedars et al. 1990). Co-therapy with the antiestrogen tamoxifen (20 mg orally daily) also limited the approximately 55% reduction usually observed after 6 months of depot goserelin to 20% in ten patients (Lumsden et al. 1987).

Until recently, leiomyomata were managed by primary surgical therapy: hysterectomy for patients whose families are complete and myomectomy for women desirous of children (Healy 1990; Matta et al. 1988). Hysterectomy is the most common surgical treatment for leiomyomata and approximately 200000 women undergo this procedure annually for fibroids in the United States alone (Esterday et al. 1983; Blumenfeld et al. 1990; Matta et al. 1988).

Since the symptomatology caused by uterine leiomyomata virtually disappears after menopause, LH-RH agonists have been successfully employed in numerous studies to induce hypoestrogenic regression of the uterine and leiomyomata volumes (Benagiano et al. 1990; Blumenfeld et al. 1990, 1991; Coddington et al. 1986; Cohen and Elia 1990; Erny et al. 1990; Friedman et al. 1987; Healy et al. 1986; Healy 1990; Heinrichs 1991; Matta et al. 1988; Perl et al. 1987; West et al. 1987). The goals of LH-RH agonist treatment of uterine leiomyomata have been to reduce the need for primary surgical therapy and to serve as a surgical adjunct, potentially reducing the operative risk, in those patients undergoing hysterectomy or myomectomy.

Most of the published studies have demonstrated a significant diminution in uterine and leiomyomata volumes of about 40% – 60% (Benagiano et al. 1990; Blumenfeld et al. 1990, 1991; Coddington et al. 1986; Cohen and Elia 1990; Erny et al. 1990; Friedman et al. 1987; Heinrichs 1991; Matta et al. 1988; Perl et al. 1987; West et al. 1987), using different modalities of drug administration intranasally, subcutaneously or by a monthly injection of a depot, slowly releasable form of an LH-RH-agonistic analog (Benagiano et al. 1990; Blumenfeld et al. 1990, 1991; Coddington et al. 1986; Cohen and Elia 1990; Erny et al. 1990; Friedman et al. 1987; Heinrichs 1991; Matta et al. 1988; Perl et al. 1987; West et al. 1987). The uterine leiomyomata have been observed to regrow in most patients several months after suspension of treatment, thus limiting the use of the LH-RH agonists in the treatment of this condition. The only serious side effect reported up to now has been a decrease of bone mineral density, which necessarily limits the duration of treatment (Mazess 1990).

Perioperative Effects

Other small studies have focused on LH-RH agonist therapy to reduce intraoperative blood loss during hysterectomy (Friedman 1989 a; Lumsden et al. 1987) or myomectomy (Friedman 1989 a), or to improve the hematologic status of anemic patients (Friedman 1989 a; Maheux et al. 1987). Postoperative febrile morbidity was also significantly reduced in a small study (Lumsden et al. 1987). The reduced blood loss (about 50%) is probably a result of the reduced pelvic blood flow found by Matta et al. (1988) and by us (Blumenfeld et al. 1991) with Doppler studies, as well as of the smaller size of tumors and the surgical incisions necessary for their excision and subsequent repair.

Pregnancy

The beneficial effect of LH-RH agonists on infertility attributed to fibroids has been reported only anecdotaly (Friedman et al. 1987; Friedman 1989 a, b; Kessel et al. 1988; Letterie et al. 1989; Lumsden et al. 1987; Matta et al. 1988; West et al. 1989; Williams and Shaw 1990). The specific examples of infertility from a cornual myoma has in two patients been in response to depot goserelin for 2 to 4 months (Gardner and Shaw 1989). A benefit of LH-RH agonist therapy for infertility from a cornual myoma was first demonstrated by Kessel et al. (1988).

Spreading the LH-RH Agonist Treatment as Repeat "On and Off" Courses

Many studies have demonstrated that administration of gonadotropin releasing-hormone agonist treatment for 6 months will produce a decrease in uterine volume in women with leiomyomata by 40% – 60% on average (Benagiano et al. 1990; Blumenfeld et al. 1990, 1991; Coddington et al. 1986; Cohen and Elia 1990; Erny et al. 1990; Friedman et al. 1987; Golan et al. 1989; Heinrichs 1991; Matta et al. 1988; Perl et al. 1987; West et al. 1987). However, relatively rapid regrowth in leiomyomata and uterine volumes occurs within 4 – 6 months after cessation of therapy to pretreatment size, a fact which limits the application and efficacy of this treatment modality as a primary medical therapy.

Maheux et al. (1985, 1987) have found that only 3 of 12 uterine leiomyomata continued to diminish in size after the first 3 months of analog treatment, all the others did not decrease, and some even augmented their volume after the first 3 of their 6 months treatment protocol. Perl et al. (1987) also concluded that 2 months of LH-RH agonist treatment may possibly be long enough to obtain a significant response in uterine volume decrease. Others (Friedman et al. 1987) have also observed the near-maximal shrinkage effect to occur by 3 months of analog therapy. Because near-maximal reduction in uterine volume was noted at 3 months of therapy, it is conceivable that a shorter treatment period than the traditional 6 months used in most previous studies, might have a less detrimental effect on bone density changes. Thus, the agonist may be best used either preoperatively as an adjunct to surgery, as suggested by Friedman et al.'s results (1989 a, b), or in women with leiomyomata who wish to temporize and postpone surgery.

However, we have decided to spread the 6 months treatment over a 12-month protocol, hoping to improve the cost-effectiveness ratio by this model of administration (Fig. 1), since (a) most of the "shrinkage effect" in the uterine and leiomyomata volumes is achieved within the first 3 months of treatment, (b) all the symptoms of abdominal heaviness, discomfort, dysmenorrhea, menometrorrhagia, or any other complaints related to the leiomyomata disappeared within the first 3 months of treatment, (c) bone resorption was significant at 6 months but insignificant at 3 months of analog treatment, (d) regrowth of the leiomyomata and uterine volumes to pretreatment size usually takes 3–6 months, and (e) the perimenopausal group of patients may need repeat drug administration until reaching their natural menopause. We have therefore undertaken an interrupted "on and off" treatment protocol of the D-6-naphthyl-alanyl-LH-RH analog (nafarelin) at a dose of 400 ug/day intranasally for 3 months, and repeat after a 3-months treatment-free period, to test the cost-effectiveness ratio in 17 premenopausal patients (Blumenfeld et al. 1991) (Figs. 2, 3).

Perimenopausal women may benefit from a short course of therapy before passing through natural menopause (Nakamura et al. 1991) and may possibly avoid operative therapy. Indeed, six of our patients (35%) reached their natural menopause, either during the 3-month drug-free interval or after the completion of the 9-month protocol. Therefore, it seems that spreading the 6-month agonist administration over a 9- to 12-month protocol does improve the cost-effectiveness ratio by gaining time and thus increasing the probability of a premenopausal patient to enter her natural menopause. This observation is in agreement with Nakamura et al.'s (1991) recent study, who demonstrated that one-third of the patients at perimenopausal age reached menopause after 16 weeks of treatment, and regrowth of leiomyomata was not observed thereafter.

A short course of therapy before natural menopause offers the possibility of treating selected patients with leiomyomata, especially perimenopausal

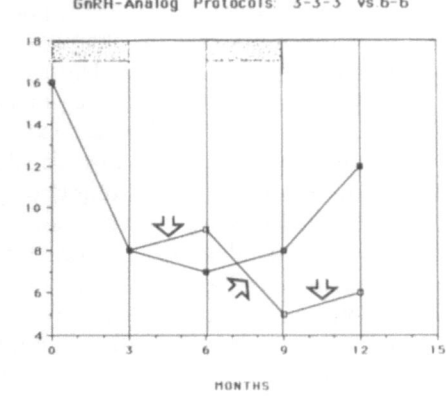

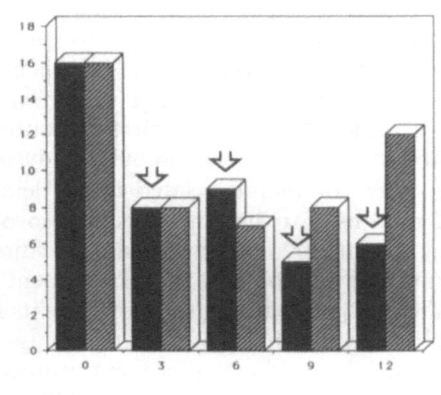

Fig. 1. A theoretical diagram of the expected decrease in uterine size (equivalent to comparable size of a pregnant uterus estimated in equivalent gestational weeks) by the traditional continuous 6 months administration of LH-RH agonists (*hatched bars*) versus the interrupted (3-3-3) on and off protocol (*black bars, arrows*)

women, thus avoiding the need for surgery. Since it is very difficult to predict precisely which patients may pass through the menopause during or immediately after a course of LH-RH agonist treatment, our interrupted, on and off protocol may increase the possibility of reaching natural menopause as compared with the continuous 6-months administration of an LH-RH-agonist, merely because the hypoestrogenic effect lasts over a longer period of time. Moreover, in those patients who have renewed bleeding and suffer from the regrowth of the fibroid uterus, a possible third, or even fourth course of 3 months of LH-RH agonist administration may be considered, each course separated from the preceding one by a 3- or 4-month drug-free interval in a "saw-teeth" manner similar to the method used in administering chemotherapeutic courses.

Since no significant bone density changes occur within the first 3 months of treatment, but may take place during 6 months of hypoestrogenism (Andreyko et al. 1988; Friedman et al. 1987; Matta et al. 1988), one may also

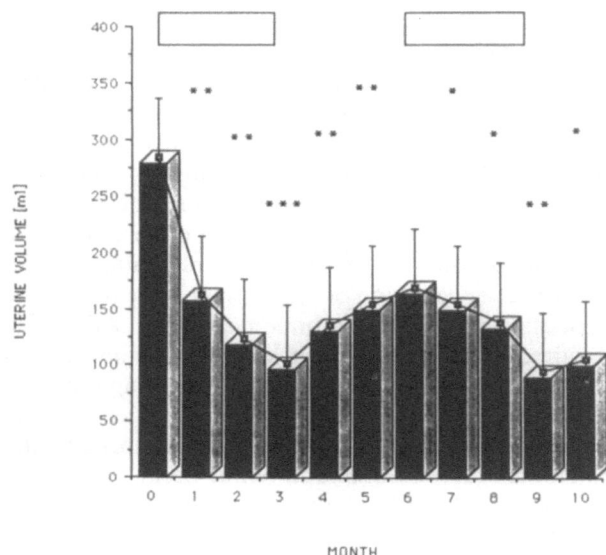

Fig. 2. Mean (± SEM) uterine volume (ml) during 10 months of on and off protocol (3-3-3) of interrupted LH-RH agonist (Nafarelin) administration to 17 women. The *rectangular horizontal bars* denote the LH-RH agonist administration periods (*, $p < 0.05$; **, $p < 0.01$; ***, $p < 0.001$)

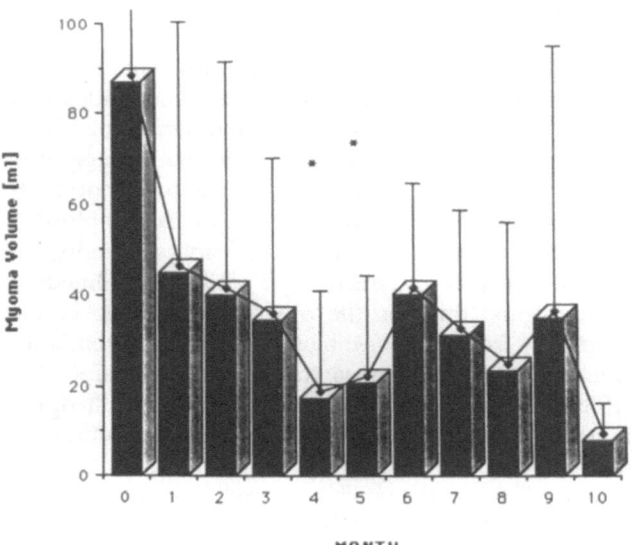

Fig. 3. Largest (mean ± SD) myoma volume (ml) during the 10 months of on and off, interrupted LH-RH agonist (Nafarelin) treatment protocol (*, $p < 0.05$)

consider this on and off protocol safer than the continuous one. In a possibly surgically high-risk patient, interrupted, on and off LH-RH agonist administration in this way may be repeated more than twice, i.e., for 18 or 24 months or as long as needed until menopause is reached. The 3-month of drug-free interval after every 3 months of agonist therapy will identify those patients who have reached menopause by showing increasing follicle-stimulating hormone (FSH) and luteinizing hormone (LH) serum levels in the presence of hypoestrogenic amenorrhea. On the other hand, those who have not reached menopause will menstruate after returning ovarian function (within 1–2 months after cessation of agonist), and are thus protected from the prolonged hypoestrogenic effect on bone resorption. Additional experience is of course required to substantiate our assumptions on the theoretic safety of multiple, repeated short-term courses of LH-RH agonists on bone metabolism. Our initial follow-up results in five of these patients within 1–3 years after completion of this on and off protocol showed normal values on dual photon X-ray of the lumbar vertebrae and femur neck.

Matta et al. (1989) have demonstrated in a longitudinal study that when buserelin was administered intranasally 400 µg three times daily to 13 premenopausal women, there was an associated small but significant reduction of 6% in their mean lumbar vertebral trabecular bone density at the end of 6 months of treatment; this loss was reversed 6 months after discontinuation of therapy (Matta et al. 1987, 1989). Our on and off protocol may provide a practical resolution to the reservations expressed by many practitioners (Matta et al. 1989) about advocating the use of LH-RH agonists in perimenopausal symptomatic women with the aim of controlling their symptoms until natural occurrence of the menopause because of the possible effect of prolonged treatment on bone metabolism.

Our findings are commensurate with a previously published report on the inverse relationship between the resistance index or the systolic to diastolic (S/D) Doppler pulsed wave ratio and uterine or leiomyoma volume (Matta et al. 1988) (Fig. 4). These observations would suggest that the reduction in size of the uterine leiomyomata is related to hypoestrogenism, possibly via the hypoestrogenic-mediated reduction in uterine blood flow. The significant reduction in blood flow may well lead to a reduction in blood loss during myomectomy or hysterectomy if performed immediately after treatment with these agents; this has the obvious advantage of minimizing postoperative morbidity from excessive bleeding, with its attendant risks of infection, adhesion formation, and need for blood transfusion. Indeed, Friedman et al.'s (1989a, b) recent randomized placebo-controlled, double-blind study found that LH-RH agonist treatment before myomectomy may decrease intraoperative blood loss.

Two of our patients who entered menopause continued to bleed and have now undergone abdominal hysterectomy to treat either a submucous or a cervical myoma. This observation of continuous bleeding in spite of hypoestrogenic levels is in agreement with other authors' experience (Friedman 1989a; Nakamura et al. 1991). Friedman (1989a) reported on three cases of

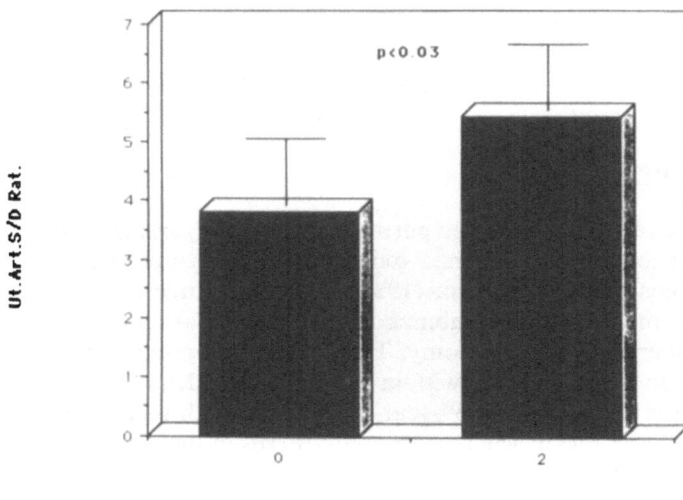

TX. MONTH

Fig. 4. Mean ± SD increase in uterine artery systolic to diastolic ratio (*Ut. Art. S/D Rat.*) within 2 months of LH-RH agonist (Nafarelin) administration to ten women with uterine leiomyomata

submucous leiomyomata with heavy vaginal bleeding during leuprolide acetate therapy, and Nakamura et al. (1991) reported on two patients with severe uterine bleeding which occurred suddenly within 6 months after menopausal status had been achieved following LH-RH agonist treatment.

Finally, in most of the published studies where the effect of LH-RH agonists on leiomyoma and uterine size was evaluated, gonadotropins and E_2 levels were measured (Andreyko et al. 1988; Benagiano et al. 1990; Blumenfeld et al. 1990; Coddington et al. 1986; Cohen and Elia 1990; Erny et al. 1990; Friedman et al. 1987; Friedman 1989 b; Gardner and Shaw 1989; Heinrichs 1991; Matta et al. 1987, 1988, 1989; Nakamura et al. 1991; West et al. 1989). E_2 levels became very low, and the gonadotropin levels also decreased, but to a relatively lesser extent than E_2 levels (Perl et al. 1987). The obvious explanation of this discrepancy lies in the difference between immunoactivity and bioactivity (Perl et al. 1987). Evans et al. (1984) reported a decrease in the ratio of bioactive to immunoreactive LH during treatment with LH-RH agonists, and suggested an alteration in LH bioactivity. It seems therefore unnecessary to measure LH and FSH concentrations every month during administration of LH-RH agonists. Serial measurements of E_2 concentrations probably reflect more accurately the gonadotropin bioactivity on the ovary. The only practical information to be gained by LH and FSH measurements is in the post-agonist treatment follow-up, to identify those patients who become menopausal and whose gonadotropin levels significantly increase.

We conclude that the interrupted on and off treatment protocol of patients with uterine leiomyomata by LH-RH agonist is more cost-effective than the continuous 6 months protocol. This interrupted protocol enables for gaining time, i.e., causing a more prolonged suppression of uterine leiomyomata without the risks of prolonged hypoestrogenic effect on bone density.

Adverse Effects

Adverse effects related particularly to leiomyomata, as opposed to those related to hypoestrogenemia generally, are related to degenerative changes (Heinrichs 1991). Friedman (1989a) reported three cases of vaginal hemorrhage from degenerating submucous myomata that required blood transfusion and emergency myomectomy. This number represents the experience from treatment of 160 women with myomata, an incidence of 1.9%. A leiomyosarcoma was identified in a 39-year-old woman with menorrhagia whose uterus was comparable in size to a pregnant uterus in the eighth gestational week. Rapid growth began between the second and third month of intranasal therapy with buserelin (Loong and Wong 1990).

Future Expectations

The impressive reduction in volume of uterine leiomyomata has been convincingly demonstrated. The mechanism of the shrinking may be attributable to changes in blood flow (Matta et al. 1988), a direct action of the agonists on the tumor (Shaw 1989), mitogens (Koutsilieris et al. 1990), or growth factors such as epidermal growth factor (Lumsden et al. 1988) or insulin-like growth factor 1 (Friedman et al. 1990).

The potentially useful clinical applications that are being evaluated include the medical adjunct to surgery in symptomatic premenopausal patients, to perimenopausal women who would benefit from shrinkage before long-term hormone replacement therapy is initiated, and infertile women with obstructive tumors of the fallopian tubes, or perhaps submucous myomata within the endometrial cavity. Even though fibroids are no longer a contraindication to low-dose oral contraception, one may be hopeful that long-term hormone replacement therapy may be safely prescribed without provoking stimulation of fibroids. Continuous progestin therapy may represent an advantageous regimen in this situation (Heinrichs 1991).

Delineation of the cohort of women with fibroids who may benefit most from LH-RH agonists therapy will require study of hematologic and hemodynamic homeostasis in relation to perioperative morbidity and the cost-effectiveness of such therapy. Some expected benefits have recently been reviewed (Heinrichs 1991; Moghissi 1990). A major impetus for LH-RH agonists therapy is the avoidance of heterologous blood transfusions for the perioperative therapy of anemic patients, and the utilization of autologous transfusions that will be possible through the control of hypermenorrhea. A further impetus will be the attempted reduction in size of uteri preoperatively so that vaginal surgery can safely replace the abdominal approach if the response is adequate. Further studies are needed to delineate more precisely the optimal duration of an LH-RH agonist treatment course, the number of courses needed and their safety, and which patients may benefit from such medical treatment instead of or in adjunct to the surgical approach.

Acknowledgement. The invaluable assistance of Mrs. Bathia Navar in preparation of this manuscript is gratefully acknowledged.

References

Andreyko JL, Blumenfeld Z, Marshall LA, Monroe SE, Hricak H, Jaffe RB (1988) Use of an agonistic analog of gonadotropin-releasing hormone (Nafarelin) to treat leiomyomata: assessment by magnetic resonance imaging. Am J Obstet Gynecol 158:903–910

Benagiano G, Morini A, Abbondante A, Aleandri V, Piccinno F, Sala D (1990) Sequential buserelin – medroxyprogesterone acetate treatment of uterine leiomyomata. In: Vickery BH, Lunenfeld B (eds) GnRH analogues in cancer and human reproduction: III. Benign and malignant tumours. Kluwer, Dordrecht, pp 53–62

Blumenfeld Z, Dirnfeld M, Beck D, Abramovici H, Brandes JM (1990) Comparison of treatment of uterine leiomyomata with 3 different GnRH agonistic analogs. In: Vickery BH, Lunenfeld B (eds) GnRH analogues in cancer and human reproduction: III. Benign and malignant tumours. Kluwer, Dordrecht, pp 45–52

Blumenfeld Z, Thaler I, Weiner Z, Beck D, Brandes JM (1991) Treatment of uterine leiomyomata with GnRH analogue (Nafarelin): a clinical protocol of interrupted (on and off) treatment. In: Lunenfeld B (ed) GnRH Analogues. Parthenon, Park Ridge, pp 43–51

Cedars MI, Lu JKH, Meldrum DR et al. (1990) Treatment of endometriosis with a long-acting gonadotropin-releasing hormone agonist plus medroxyprogesterone acetate. Obstet Gynecol 75:641

Coddington CC, Collins RL, Shawker TH, Anderson R, Loriaux DL, Winkel CA (1986) Long-acting gonadotropin hormone-releasing hormone analog used to treat uteri. Fertil Steril 45:624–629

Cohen J, Elia D (1990) Relevance of an LHRH agonist to the treatment of uterine fibromyomas. In: Vickey BH, Lunenfeld B (eds) GnRH analogues in cancer and human reproduction: III. Benign and malignant tumours. Kluwer, Dordrecht, pp 33–44

Donnez J, Schrurs B, Gillerot S, Sandow J, Clerckx F (1989) Treatment of uterine fibroids with implants of gonadotropin-releasing hormone agonist: assessment by hysterography. Fertil Steril 51:947

Erny R, Milliet E, Boubli L (1990) Treatment of uterine fibroids with intra-nasal buserelin. In: Vickery BH, Lunenfeld B (eds) GnRH analogues in cancer and human reproduction: III. Benign and malignant tumours. Kluwer, Dordrecht, pp 21–26

Esterday CL, Grimes DA, Riggs JA (1983) Hysterectomy in the United States. Obstet Gynecol 62:203–220

Evans RM, Doelle GC, Lindner J, Bradley V, Rabın D (1984) An LHRH agonist decreases biologic activity and modified chromatographic behavior of LH in man. J Clin Invest 73:262–270

Filcori M, Hall DA, Laughlin JS, Rivier J, Vale W, Crowley WF (1983) A conservative approach to the management of uterine leiomyomata: pituitary desensitization by a luteinizing hormone releasing hormone analogue. Am J Obstet Gynecol 147:726–729

Friedman AJ (1989 a) Vaginal hemorrhage associated with degenerating submucous leiomyoma during leuprolide acetate treatment. Fertil Steril 52:152

Friedman AJ (1989 b) Treatment of leiomyomata uteri with short-term leuprolide followed by leuprolide plus estrogen-progestin hormone replacement therapy for 2 years: a pilot study. Fertil Steril 51:526

Friedman AJ (1990) Advances in the treatment of leiomyomata uteri with leuprolide. In: Vickery BH, Lunenfeld B (eds) GnRH analogues in cancer and human reproduction: III. Benign and malignant tumours. Kluwer, Dordrecht, pp 27–32

Friedman AJ, Barbieri RL, Benaceraff BR, Schiff I (1987) Treatment of leiomyomata with intranasal or subcutaneous leuprolide, a gonadotropin releasing-hormone agonist. Fertil Steril 48: 560–564

Friedman AJ, Barbieri RL, Doubilet PM, Fine C, Schiff I (1988) A randomized, double-blind trial of a gonadotroph releasing-hormone agonist (leuprolide) with or without medroxy-progesterone acetate in the treatment of leiomyomata uteri. Fertil Steril 49: 404–409

Friedman AJ, Harrison-Atlas D, Barbieri RL, Benacerraf B, Gleason R, Schiff I (1989 a) A randomized, placebo-controlled, double-blind study evaluating the efficacy of leuprolide acetate depot in the treatment of uterine leiomyomata. Fertil Steril 51: 251

Friedman AJ, Rein MS, Harrison-Atlas D, Garfield JM, Doubilet PM (1989 b) A random-ized, placebo-controlled, double-blind study evaluating leuprolide acetate depot treat-ment before myomectomy. Fertil Steril 52: 728–733

Friedman AJ, Rein MS, Pandian MR, Barbieri RL (1990) Fasting serum growth hormone and insulin-like growth factor-I and -II concentrations in women with leiomyomata uteri treated with leuprolide acetate or placebo. Fertil Steril 53: 250

Gardner RL, Shaw RW (1989) Cornual fibroids: a conservative approach to restoring tubal potency using a gonadotropin-releasing hormone agonist (goserelin) with successful pregnancy. Fertil Steril 52: 332

George M, L'Homme C, Lefort J, Gras C, Comarn-Schally AM, Schally AV (1989) Long-term use of an LH-RH agonist in the management of uterine leiomyomas: a study of 17 cases. Int J Fertil 34: 19

Golan A, Bukovsky I, Schneider D et al. (1989) D-Trp⁶-luteinizing hormone-releasing hor-mone microcapsules in the treatment of uterine leiomyomas. Fertil Steril 52: 406

Healy DL (1990) The use of LH-RH analogues in the treatment of uterine fibroids. In: Vickery BH, Lunenfeld B (eds) GnRH analogues in cancer and human reproduction: III. Benign and malignant tumours. Kluwer, Dordrecht, pp 1–20

Healy DL, Fraser HM, Lawson SL (1984) Shrinkage of a uterine fibroid after subcutaneous infusion of a LH-RH agonist. BMJ 289: 1267

Healy DL, Lawson SR, Abbott M, Baird DT, Fraser HM (1986) Toward removing uterine fibroids without surgery: subcutaneous infusion of a luteinizing-hormone releasing hor-mone agonist commencing in the luteal phase. J Clin Endocrinol Metab 63: 619–624

Heinrichs WL (1991) Gonadotropin releasing-hormone agonists (GnRH-a) in gynecological practice: endometriosis and leiomyomata uteri. In: Mishell DR, Kirshbaum TH, Mor-row CP (eds) Yearbook of obstetrics and gynecology. Mosby, St. Louis, p 333

Kessel B, Liu J, Mortola J, Berger S, Yen SS (1988) Treatment of uterine fibroids with agonist analogs of gonadotropin-releasing hormone. Fertil Steril 49: 538

Koutsilieris M, Michand J, Mikolis A (1990) Preferential mitogenic activity for myoblast-like cells can be extracted from uterine leiomyomata tissues. Am J Obstet Gynecol 163: 1665

Letterie GS, Coddington CC, Winkel CA, Shawker TH, Loriaux DL, Collins RL (1989) Efficacy of a gonadotropin-releasing hormone agonist in the treatment of uterine leiomy-omata: long-term follow-up. Fertil Steril 51: 951

Loong EPL, Wong FWS (1990) Uterine leiomyosarcoma diagnosed during treatment with agonist hormone-releasing hormone for presumed uterine fibroid. Fertil Steril 54: 530

Lumsden MA, West CP, Baird DT (1987) Goserelin therapy before surgery for uterine fibroids. Lancet 1: 36

Lumsden MA, West CP, Bramley T, Rumgay L, Baird DT (1988) The binding of epidermal growth factor to the human uterus and leiomyomata in women rendered hypoestrogenic by continuous administration of an LH-RH agonist. Br J Obstet Gynaecol 95: 1299

Maheux R, Guilloteau C, Lemay A, Bastide A, Fazekas AIA (1985) Luteinizing hormone-re-leasing hormone agonist and uterine leiomyoma: a pilot study. Am J Obstet Gynecol 152: 1034–1038

Maheux R, Lemay A, Merat P (1987) Use of intranasal luteinizing hormone-releasing hormone agonist in uterine leiomyomas. Fertil Steril 47: 229–233

Maheux R, Lemay A, Turcot-Lemay L (1988) Dose-related inhibition of acute luteinizing hormone response during luteinizing hormone-releasing hormone agonist treatment of uterine leiomyomata. Am J Obstet Gynecol 158:361

Matta WH, Shaw RW, Hesp R, Katz D (1987) Hypogonadism induced by luteinizing hormone-releasing hormone agonist analogues: effect on bone density in premenopausal women. BMJ 294:1523–1528

Matta WHM, Stabile I, Shaw RW, Campbell S (1988) Doppler assessment of uterine blood flow changes in patients with fibroids receiving the gonadotropin-releasing hormone agonist buserelin. Fertil Steril 49:1083–1085

Matta WHM, Shaw RW, Nye M (1989) Long-term follow-up of patients with uterine fibroids after treatment with the LH-RH agonist buserelin. Br J Obstet Gynaecol 96:200–206

Mazess R (1990) Bone densiometry of the axial skeleton. Orthop Clin North Am 21:51

McLachlan RI, Healy DL, Burger HG (1986) Clinical aspects of LH-RH analogues in gynecology: a review. Br J Obstet Gynaecol 93:431–446

Moghissi K (1990) Gonadotropin releasing hormones: clinical applications in gynecology. J Reprod Med 35:1097

Nakamura Y, Yoshimura Y, Yamada H, Ubukata Y, Ando M, Suzuki M (1991) Treatment of uterine leiomyomata with a luteinizing hormone-releasing hormone agonist: the possibility of nonsurgical management in selected perimenopausal women. Fertil Steril 55:900–905

Perl V, Leal O, Marquez J, Zacharias S, Schally AV, Gomezu-Lira C, Comaru-Schally AM (1987) Treatment of leiomyomata uteri with [D-TRP6]-luteinizing hormone-releasing hormone. Fertil Steril 48:383–389

Ross RK, Pike NC, Vessey NP, Bull D, Yates D, Casagrande JT (1986) Risk factors for uterine fibroids: reduced risk associated with oral contraceptives. BMJ 293:359–364

Schlaff WD, Zerhouni EA, Huth JAM, Chen J, Damewood MD, Rock JA (1989) A placebo-controlled trial of a depot gonadotropin-releasing hormone analogue (leuprolide) in the treatment of uterine leiomyomata. Obstet Gynecol 74:856–862

Shaw RW (1989) Mechanism of LH-RH analogue action in uterine fibroids. Horm Res 32:150

Soules MR, McCarty KS (1982) Leiomyomas: steroid receptor content. Am J Obstet Gynecol 143:6–13

Spellacy WN, Lemaire WJ, Buhl WC, Birk SA, Bradley BA (1972) Plasma growth hormone and estradiol levels in women with uterine myomas. Obstet Gynecol 40:829–837

Tamaya T, Fujimoto J, Okada H (1985) Comparison of cellular levels of steroid receptors in uterine leiomyoma and myometrium. Acta Obstet Gynecol Scand 64:307–314

Van Leusden HAIM (1986) Rapid reduction of uterine myomas after short term treatment with microencapsulated D-Trp6-LH-RH. Lancet 1:213

Van Leusden HAIM (1988) Triptorelin to prevent hysterectomy in patients with leiomyomas. Lancet 2:508

Van der Spuy ZM, Fieggan AG, Wood MJA, Pienaar CA (1989) The short-term use of luteinizing hormone-releasing hormone analogues in uterine fibroids. Horm Res [Suppl 1]:137–140

Vollenhoven BJ, Shekleton P, McDonald J, Healy DL (1990) Clinical predictors for buserelin acetate treatment of uterine fibroids: a prospective study of 40 women. Fertil Steril 54:1032–1038

West CP, Williamson J, Lumsden MA, Baird DT, Lawson S (1987) Shrinkage of uterine fibroids during therapy with goserelin (Zoladex): a luteinizing hormone-releasing hormone agonist administered as a monthly subcutaneous depot. Fertil Steril 48:45–51

West CP, Lumsden MA, Baird DT (1989) LH-RH analogues and fibroids-potential for longer-term use. Horm Res 32:146

Wilson EA, Yang F, Rees ED (1980) Estradiol and progesterone binding in uterine leiomyomata and in normal uterine tissues. Obstet Gynecol 55:20–27

Williams IA, Shaw RW (1990) Effect of nafarelin on uterine fibroids measured by ultrasound and magnetic resonance imaging. Eur J Obstet Gynecol Reprod Biol 34:111

On the Management of Metastatic Prostate Cancer with LH-RH Analogs

J. H. M. Blom and F. H. Schröder

Department of Urology, Erasmus University, Dr. Molewaterplein 40, 3015 GD Rotterdam, The Netherlands

With the availability of luteinizing hormone releasing hormone (LH-RH) agonists, and in the future of maybe also of LH-RH antagonists, new principles were introduced into the clinical management of human prostate carcinoma and other steroid-hormone-dependent tumors (Schröder et al. 1987). LH-RH agonists offered a new principle of suppressing testicular androgen to castration levels, the major advantage of which over the classical forms of treatment with estrogen administration or castration seemed to be an absence of physical side effects and a reduction of physiological side effects. For these advantages a much higher price has to be paid, and it now remains questionable in how far LH-RH agonists will be able to compete with other principles of castration in the management of this disease.

This situation would change immediately, and medical reasoning would urge the use of LH-RH agonists if other advantages of this treatment principle could be demonstrated. There are currently no data that document a direct effect of the decapeptides on prostatic carcinoma cells. Another potential development, along with the developments of LH-RH and other peptide hormone agonists, is the facilitation of combination treatment of human prostate carcinoma using various drugs. Many clinical efforts have been made worldwide to prove or disprove the theory that simultaneous testicular and adrenal androgen suppression is a superior form of management of prostate carcinoma than testicular androgen suppression alone. The controversy surrounding this point was initiated by Labrie and his coworkers (1983). Contributory evidence will be discussed in this chapter. Recent evidence shows that aromatase inhibition (Manni et al. 1986), somatotropin analogs, and some cytostatic drugs (Jones et al. 1986) exert some degree of tumor control in metastatic prostate cancer. Combinations of such treatment principles may allow control to be exerted over hormone-dependent *and* hormone-independent cell populations, the latter being responsible for the death of the patients.

A large volume of literature, which includes reports on a number of randomized studies comparing LH-RH-analogs with standard forms of treatment, has appeared without demonstrating any significant differences in treatment results. These include the papers by the Leuprolide Study Group (1984), Roger et al. (1985), Parmar et al. (1985 and 1987), Koutsilieris et al. (1986), Schröder et al. (1987), and Debruyne (1989).

Depot Preparations

Most of the LH-RH agonists initially required daily administration either by subcutaneous injections or by intranasal sprays. This led to potential problems in patient compliance, especially in elderly men. To minimize the difficulties relating to administration, implant preparations of the LH-RH agonists have been developed. The most well-known implant preparation is the monthly injectable subcutaneous depot preparation goserelin (Zoladex). Several studies have demonstrated the clinical efficacy and safety of this treatment formulation (Grant et al. 1986; Debruyne et al. 1988; Kotake et al. 1988; Mauriac et al. 1988; Alcini et al. 1988; Metz et al. 1988). Parmar and associates (1985, 1987), Roger and coworkers (1985), and De Sy and coworkers (1986) reported favourable results with the intramuscularly injectable depot preparation D-Trp^6-LH-RH (decapeptyl). Recently the Leuprolide Study Group has published their results on a monthly depot preparation of leuprolide (Sharifi et al. 1990), showing that this depot formulation is as effective and safe as the daily injectable formulation.

The first clinical use of a depot buserelin was described by Waxman and coworkers (1986). In our clinic, a study was carried out in 1987 and 1988 to compare the pharmacokinetics and the endocrinological effects of a monthly and a 2-monthly subcutaneous depot preparation of buserelin in 14 patients with metastatic prostate cancer (Blom et al. 1989). It was shown that a 2-monthly preparation of buserelin was as equally effective as the monthly preparation in suppressing plasma testosterone to castration levels.

Monthly and 2-monthly, and maybe in the future even longer-lasting, preparations of LH-RH agonists provide the opportunity of a safe and effective treatment of advanced prostate cancer with optimal comfort for the patient, which results in a better patient compliance.

Flare Phenomenon

The mechanism of action of LH-RH agonists stems from a superstimulation of the pituitary, ultimately resulting in downregulation of the LH-RH receptors and leading to a refractory condition of anterior pituitary cells to LH-RH secretion (Sandow and Beier 1985). This process occurs over a 1- to 3-week period, during which time there may be supersecretion of both luteinizing hormone (LH) and testosterone. Administration of LH-RH agonists to patients with metastatic prostate carcinoma has been associated with an apparent transient tumor stimulation, manifested by increases in acid phosphatase levels and skeletal pain in up to 10% of patients (Schulze and Senge 1990). This flare phenomenon may even lead to the sudden death of the patient (Thompson et al. 1990). The clinical symptoms, caused by the initial rise of plasma testosterone levels in the first weeks of LH-RH agonist treatment can be prevented by administering antiandrogens or diethylstilbestrol (DES) during this early period (Mahler and Denis 1988; Denis 1989).

Influence of Different Antiandrogens on Flare

The question arises as to whether all antiandrogens are equally effective in preventing flare symptoms. Waxman and coworkers (1988) studied the endocrinological effects of two different dose regimens of cyproterone acetate (CPA) and flutamide in the prevention of tumor flare. They found that both dose regimens of CPA (50 mg t.i.d. and 100 mg t.i.d.) were able to prevent testosterone from rising above the baseline value after injection of a depot preparation of buserelin, but that flutamide (250 mg t.i.d.) failed to do so. They based their conclusions mainly on plasma testosterone levels, however, and not on tumor markers such as prostate acid phosphatase or prostate specific antigen. Clinical symptoms deteriorated in this early phase of treatment in three of eight patients who received 50 mg CPA t.i.d. and in one of eight patients who received flutamide.

Schulze and Senge (1990) studied 21 patients with previously untreated metastatic prostate cancer. They randomly assigned these 21 patients to four treatment groups. In the first group five patients were treated with the LH-RH agonist goserelin (Zoladex) alone. In the second group six patients were treated with Zoladex plus the steroidal antiandrogen CPA, starting 7 days before the initial Zoladex injection. In the third group five patients were treated with Zoladex plus the nonsteroidal antiandrogen flutamide; the flutamide therapy was started 1 day before the initial Zoladex injection. In the fourth group, five patients were treated with Zoladex plus flutamide, but the flutamide treatment was begun 7 days before the initial Zoladex injection.

As might be expected, there was an initial rise in plasma LH and testosterone levels in all four treatment groups. This rise was accompanied by a rise in serum prostatic acid phosphatase in group 1 and group 3 only. In group 2 and group 4, this rise in serum prostatic acid phosphatase did not occur. It was concluded that, at least from an endocrinological viewpoint, the steroidal antiandrogen CPA was as effective as the nonsteroidal antiandrogen flutamide. Starting this adjuvant therapy only 1 day prior to Zoladex injection was ineffective in preventing the biochemical flare. The nonsteroidal antiandrogen nilutamide (Anandron) is also capable of preventing the adverse effects of the flare phenomenon (Kuhn et al., 1989).

Testicular Impairment

One of the possible advantages of treatment with LH-RH agonists seemed to be the reversibility of testicular functions after discontinuation of therapy. It may be possible to decide to stop hormonal therapy and start other treatment modalities once the tumor has become hormone independent. The advantage would be that the patient could recover his sexual functions. Several observations, however, cast doubt on this assumption. It has been shown that LH-RH agonists cause a LH receptor loss in the Leydig cell and that they exert a direct action on receptors for the Sertoli cell peptides on the Leydig cell (Sandow and Beier 1985). Petersson and coworkers (1987) observed a significant decrease in the conversion mediated by the enzymes 3β-hydroxysteroid dehydrogenase, 17α-hydroxylase, and C_{17-20} lyase under treatment with the LH-RH agonist Zoladex in nine patients with prostate carcinoma. This observation indicated that LH-RH agonists act not only at the pituitary level, but also at the testicular level. It is, however, unclear whether this effect is reversible or not.

Decensi and coworkers (1989) studied 14 patients with prostatic cancer who were being treated with a slow-release LH-RH agonist for a median of 21 months. They found that the plasma testosterone response to human chorionic gonadotropin (HCG) was markedly reduced in most of the patients. Administration of 5000 IU HCG resulted in a median rise of plasma testosterone from 0.25 to 1.65 nmol/l. A second HCG test was repeated in five patients, 6 months after discontinuation of treatment. Median plasma testosterone levels were found to have increased to a maximum of 2.6 nmol/l, compared to 28.2 nmol/l in an age-matched control group ($p = 0.008$). Their conclusion was that gonadal impairment after long-term treatment with LH-RH agonists may not be as reversible as is generally suggested.

Total Androgen Suppression

It is still controversial whether treatment with an LH-RH agonist or orchiectomy alone is equally effective as the combination of an LH-RH agonist and an antiandrogen or DES. Several studies have tried to give a definitive solution to this controversy. The first observation that total androgen blockade might be superior to testicular androgen suppression alone came from Labrie and his coworkers (1983). In later reports they extended their experience (1985, 1986). Crawford and coworkers (1989) conducted a randomized study in 603 previously untreated patients with disseminated prostate cancer. They compared the clinical efficacy of the combination of the LH-RH agonist leuprolide and the antiandrogen flutamide with the clinical effects of leuprolide and a placebo. They observed longer progression-free survival in the group of 303 patients receiving leuprolide and flutamide (16.5 versus 13.9 months; $p = 0.039$) than in the 300 patients who received leuprolide plus placebo. They also observed an increase in the median length of survival (35.6 versus 28.3 months; $p = 0.035$) in the group of patients treated with complete androgen blockade. They concluded that the treatment with leuprolide and flutamide was superior to leuprolide alone in patients with advanced prostate cancer.

Several investigators were unable to reproduce these results. In two separate multicenter studies, Schröder and coworkers (1987) compared the endocrine parameters, the rate and duration of response, and the rate of progression in 58 patients who were treated with the LH-RH agonist buserelin alone and in 13 patients who were treated with a combination of buserelin and CPA. The endocrine studies showed an effective suppression of plasma testosterone to castration levels in both treatment groups. Response did not differ between the two treatment groups, nor did the rate of progression. A superiority of total androgen suppression could not be demonstrated. In a prospective randomized study, Denis and coworkers (1990) compared the clinical efficacy of the combination of the LH-RH agonist Zoladex and the antiandrogen flutamide with the clinical efficacy of orchiectomy alone in 327 patients with metastatic prostate cancer. They found that the combination of Zoladex and flutamide significantly delayed the time to progression as compared with orchiectomy. However, no difference in survival could be detected. Thus, a delay in the appearance of progression did not result in improved survival. Iversen and coworkers (1990) were also unable to demonstrate any significant clinical superiority of the combination of Zoladex and flutamide over orchiectomy in a randomized phase III trial of 264 patients. More reports confirm this observation, such as the study by Schulze and coworkers (1987). Although there are an increasing number of reports on this subject, the controversy as to whether total androgen blockade is superior to testicular androgen suppression still remains unanswered.

Discussion

The actual rate of progression of 40% at 12 months under endocrine management observed in the study of Schröder and coworkers (1987) confirms other observations and indicates once again that the fate of patients with metastatic prostate carcinoma is ultimately determined by the hormone-independent cell population present in this malignancy. In dealing with hormone-dependent prostate cancer, the question of whether very small amounts of circulating androgens such as the plasma levels in humans after castration are sufficient to stimulate growth of the tumor is not at present entirely resolved. Much information from various experimental models is available, but some of it is contradictory. The ultimate answer will have to come from well-controlled clinical trials, which must then show a clear-cut advantage of the combination treatment using a principle that achieves a castration effect together with a drug that counteracts or inhibits the production of adrenal androgens. Some of the criticism that can be advanced against the data of Labrie and coworkers includes the phase II character of the data presented, the use of weak response criteria, the use of historical comparisons without establishing the comparability of the groups of patients involved, and the inclusion of the stable disease category as a responding group in statistical analysis. The data presented in the paper by Schröder and coworkers contradict the data of Labrie and his group in that they show high progression rates for the total androgen suppression group. However, patient numbers are too small, and the study conducted was not a prospective randomized trial. Such a study has, however, been concluded by the EORTC GU group. Preliminary results were published by Robinson and Hetherington (1986). Protocol 30805 compares orchiectomy to orchiectomy plus CPA (150 mg per day) and to DES (1 mg per day) in 241 patients with metastasized prostate carcinoma who were equally randomized to the three treatment modalities. No difference in the rate of progression or in survival resulted between the three groups.

An interesting aspect is that since publication of the report by Shearer et al. (1973), 1 mg DES is known not to completely suppress plasma testosterone to castration levels. Plasma testosterone levels with 1 mg DES daily are in the range of 60–80 ng/100 ml. Two randomized studies in France comparing standard therapy with a combination of an LH-RH agonist and the potent antiandrogen Anandron (nilutamide) did not show a difference in progression rates either (Navratil 1987; Brisset et al. 1987). Possibly, the combination treatment may be superior as far as early response is concerned.

For the interpretation of the EORTC study 30805, the important question is whether CPA is effective in suppressing adrenal androgens. Discussions on this problem have been published by Poyet and Labrie (1985) and Habenicht et al. (1986). The classical experiments using the weight of the ventral prostate of the rat as a model in castrated and androgen-supplemented animals remain most important and informative for determining the effectiveness and potency of an antiandrogen. The study by Neri et al. (1972) using flutamide and CPA, "each administered at a constant dose (10 mg/kg) concurrently with testosterone propionate over a wide dose range reveals that Sch 13521 (Flutamide) was equipotent to cyproterone acetate as an antiandrogen." The effectiveness of CPA in suppressing acid phosphatase activity in prostate cancer patients during testosterone peak in the initial treatment phase with an LH-RH-agonist shows this drug to be effective in the human situation, too.

The fact that the group receiving 1 mg DES treatment in the EORTC protocol 30805 did not show a significant difference in the rate of progression compared with the group receiving castration and the combination treatment in this study suggests that even the achievement of castration levels of plasma testosterone is not crucial in the management of this tumor. It is not currently known at what level plasma testosterone will become stimulating in the clinical situation. The available data, however, suggest that, in agreement with observations reported by Oesterling et al. (1986), the adult human prostate and prostate carcinoma are not usually stimulated by tissue levels resulting from castration levels of plasma testosterone.

References

Alcini E, D'Addessi A, Destito A, Grasso G (1988) LH-RH analogue treatment for advanced prostate cancer. Am J Clin Oncol 11 [Suppl 2]:S120–S122

Blom JHM, Hirdes WH, Schröder FH, De Jong FH, Kwekkeboom DJ, van 't Veen AJ, Sandow J, Krauss B (1989) Pharmacokinetics and endocrine effects of the LHRH analogue buserelin after subcutaneous implantation of a slow release preparation in prostatic cancer patients. Urol Res 17:43–46

Brisset J-M, Boccon-Gibod L, Botto H, Camey M, Cariou G, Duclos J-M, Duval F, Gonties D, Jorest R, Lamy L, LeDuc A, Mouton A, Petit M, Prawerman A, Richard F, Savatovsky I, Vallancie G (1987) Anandron (RU 23908) associated to surgical castration in previously untreated stage D prostate cancer: a multicenter comparative study of two doses of the drug and of a placebo. In: Khoury S, Murphy GP (eds) Cancer of the prostate. Liss, New York

Crawford ED, Eisenberger MA, McLeod DG, Spaulding JT, Benson R, Dorr FA, Blumenstein BA, Davis MA, Goodman PJ (1989) A controlled trial of leuprolide with and without flutamide in prostatic carcinoma. N Engl J Med 321:419–424

Debruyne F (1989) Luteinizing hormone-releasing hormone analogues alone in the treatment of advanced disease. Horm Res 32 [Suppl 1]:62–65

Debruyne FMJ, Denis L, Lunglmayr G, Mahler C, Newling DWW, Richards B, Robinson MRG, Smith PH, Weil EHJ, Whelan P (1988) Long-term therapy with a depot luteinizing hormone analogue (Zoladex) in patients with advanced prostatic carcinoma. J Urol 140:775–777

Denis L (1989) LHRH analogues in combination with an anti-androgen in the treatment of advanced disease. Horm Res 32 [Suppl 1]:66–68

Denis L, Keuppens F, Robinson M, Mahler C, Smith P, Pinto de Carvalho APA, Newling D, Bono A, Sylvester R, De Pauw M, Vermeylen K, Ongena P and members of the EORTC GU group (1990) Complete androgen blockade: data from an EORTC 30853 trial. Sem Urol 8:166–174

Decensi AU, Guarneri D, Marroni P, Di Cristina L, Paganuzzi M, Boccardo F (1989) Evidence for testicular impairment after long-term treatment with a luteinizing hormone-releasing hormone agonist in elderly men. J Urol 142:1235–1238

De Sy WA, De Meyer JM, Casselman J, De Smet R, Renders G, Schelfhout W, De Wilde P (1986) A comparative study of a long acting luteinizing hormone releasing hormone agonist (decapeptyl) and orchiectomy in the treatment of advanced prostatic cancer. Acta Urol Belg 54:221–229

Grant JBF, Ahmed SR, Shalte SM, Costello CB, Howell A, Blacklock NJ (1986) Testosterone and gonadotrophin profiles in patients on daily or monthly LHRH analogue ICI 118630 (Zoladex) compared with orchiectomy. Br J Urol 58:539–544

Habenicht UF, Witthaus E, Neumann F (1986) Antiandrogens and LH-RH agonists endocrinology in the initial phase of their use. Akt Urol 17:10–16

Iversen P, Christensen MG, Friis E, Hornbøl P, Hvidt V, Iversen HG, Klarskov P, Krarup T, Lund F, Mogensen P, Pedersen T, Rasmussen F, Rose C, Skaarup P, Wolf H (1990) A phase III trial of Zoladex and Flutamide versus orchiectomy in the treatment of patients with advanced carcinoma of the prostate. Cancer 66:1058–1066

Jones WG, Fosså SD, Bono A, Croles JJ, Stoter G, De Pauw M, Sylvester R, members of the EORTC Gentourinary Tract Cancer Cooperative Group (1986) Mitimycin-C in the treatment of metastatic prostate cancer: report on an EORTC phase II study. World J Urol 4:182–185

Kotake T, Usami M, Sonoda T, Matsuda M, Okajima E, Osafune M, Isurugi K, Akaza H, Saitoh Y (1988) LH-RH agonist, Zoladex (Goserelin), depot formulation in the treatment of prostatic cancer. Am J Clin Oncol 11 [Suppl 2]:S108–S111

Koutsilieris M, Faure N, Tolis G, Laroche B, Robert G, Ackman CFD (1986) Objective response and disease outcome in 59 patients with stage D_2 prostatic cancer treated with either buserelin or orchiectomy. Urology 27:221–228

Kuhn J-M, Billebaud T, Navratil H, Moulonguet A, Fiet J, Grise P, Louis J-F, Costa P, Husson J-M, Dahan R, Bertagna C, Edelstein R (1989) Prevention of the transient edverse effects of a gonadotropin-releasing hormone analogue (buserelin) in metastatic prostatic carcinoma by administration of an antiandrogen (nilutamide). N Engl J Med 321:413–418

Labrie F, Dupont A, Belanger A, Lacoursiere Y, Raynaud JP, Husson JM, Gareau J, Fazekas ATA, Sandow J, Monfette G, Girard JG, Emond J, Houle JG (1983) New approach in the treatment of prostate cancer: complete instead of partial withdrawal of androgens. Prostate 4:579–594

Labrie F, Dupont A, Belanger A (1985) Combination therapy with flutamide and castration (LHRH agonist or orchiectomy) in advanced prostate cancer: a marked improvement in response and survival. J Steroid Biochem 23:833–841

Labrie F, Dupont A, Belanger A, St-Arnaud R, Giguere M, Lacoursiere Y, Emond J, Monfette G (1986) Treatment of prostate cancer with gonadotropin-relasing hormone agonists. Endocr Rev 7:67–74

Leuprolide Study Group (1984) Leuprolide versus Diethylstilbestrol for metastatic prostate cancer. N Engl J Med 311:1281–1286

Mahler C, Denis L (1988) Simultaneous administration of a luteinizing hormone releasing hormone agonist and diethylstilbestrol in the initial treatment of prostatic cancer. Am J Clin Oncol 11 [Suppl 2]:S127–S128

Manni A, Santen RJ, Boucher AE, Lipton A, Harvey H, Simmonds M, White-Hershey D, Gordon RA, Rohner T, Drago J (1986) Hormone stimulation and chemotherapy in advanced prostate cancer: interim analysis of an ongoing randomized trial. Anticancer Res 6:309–314

Mauriac L, Coste P, Richaud P, Lamarche P, Mage P, Bonichon F (1988) Clinical study of an LH-RH agonist (ICI 118630, Zoladex) in the treatment of prostatic cancer. Am J Clin Oncol 11 [Suppl 2]:S117–S119

Metz R, Namer M, Adenis L, Audhuy B, Bugat R, Colombel P, Couette JE, Grise P, Khater R, LePorz B, Levin G, Marti P, Mauriac M, Rouxel A, Tetelboum R (1988) Zoladex as primary therapy in advanced prostatic cancer. Am J Clin Oncol 11 [Suppl 2]:S112–S114

Navratil H (1987) Double-blind study of Anandron versus placebo in Stage D2 prostate cancer patients receiving buserelin. Results in 49 cases from a multicentre study. In: Khoury S, Murphy GP (eds) Cancer of the prostate. Liss, New York

Neri R, Florance K, Koziol P, Van Cleave S (1972) A biological profile of a nonsteroidal antiandrogen, Sch 13521 (4'-nitro-3'-trifluoromethylisobutyranalide). Endocrinology 91:427–437

Oesterling JE, Epstein JI, Walsh PC (1986) The inability of adrenal androgens to stimulate the adult human prostate: an autopsy evaluation of men with hypogonadotropic hypogonadism and panhypopituitarism. J Urol 136:1030–1034

Parmar H, Lightman SL, Allen L, Phillips RH, Edwards L, Schally AV (1985) Randomised controlled study of orchiectomy vs long-acting D-Trp[6]-LHRH microcapsules in advanced prostatic carcinoma. Lancet 30:1201–1205

Parmar H, Edwards L, Phillips RH, Allen L, Lightman SL (1987) Orchiectomy versus long-acting D-Trp[6]-LHRH in advanced prostatic cancer. Br J Urol 59:248–254

Petersson F, Hammar M, Mathson K, Hjertberg H, Varenhorst E (1987) Influence of continuous luteinizing hormone-releasing hormone agonist on steroidogenic enzymes in the human testis. Scand J Urol Nephrol 21:267–271

Poyet P, Labrie F (1985) Comparison of the antiandrogenic/androgenic activities of flutamide, cyproterone actetate and megestrol acetate. Mol Cell Endocrinol 42:283–288

Robinson MRG, Hetherington J (1986) The EORTC studies: is there an optimal endocrine management for M1 prostatic cancer? World J Urol 4:171–175

Roger M, Duchier J, Lahlou N, Nahoul K, Schally AV (1985) Treatment of prostatic carcinoma with D-Trp[6]-LH-RH: plasma hormone levels after daily subcutaneous injections and periodic administration of delayed-release preparations. Prostate 7:271–282

Sandow J, Beier B (1985) LHRH agonists: mechanism of action and effect on target tissues. Prog Clin Biol Res 185A:121–142

Schröder FH, Lock TMTW, Chadha DR, Debruyne FMJ, Karthaus HFM, De Jong FH, Klijn JGM, Matroos AW, De Voogt HJ (1987) Metastatic cancer of the prostate managed with buserelin versus buserelin plus cyproterone acatate. J Urol 137:912–918

Schulze H, Senge T (1990) Influence of different types of antiandrogens on luteinizing hormone-releasing hormone analogue-induced testosterone surge in patients with metastatic carinoma of the prostate. J Urol 144:934–941

Schulze H, Isaacs J, Senge T (1987) Inability of complete androgen blockade to increase survival of patients with advanced prostatic cancer as compared to standard hormonal therapy. J Urol 137:909–911

Sharifi R, Soloway M, The Leuprolide Study Group (1990) Clinical study of leuprolide depot formulation in the treatment of advanced prostate cancer. J Urol 143:68–71

Shearer RJ, Hendry WF, Sommerville IF, Fergusson JD (1973) Plasma testosterone: an accurate monitor of hormone treatment in prostatic cancer. Br J Urol 45:668–677

Thompson IM, Zeidman EJ, Rodriguez FR (1990) Sudden death due to disease flare with luteinizing hormone-releasing hormone agonist therapy for carcinoma of the prostate. J Urol 144:1479–1480

Waxman JH, Sandow J, Man A, Barnett MJ, Hendry WF, Besser GM, Oliver RTD, Magill PJ (1986) The first clinical use of depot buserelin for advanced prostatic carcinoma. Cancer Chemother Pharmacol 18:174–175

Waxman J, Williams G, Sandow J, Hewitt G, Abel P, Farah N, Fleming J, Cox J, O'Donoghue EPN, Sikora K (1988) The clinical and endocrine assessment of three different antiandrogen regimens combined with a very long-acting gonadotrophin-releasing hormone analogue. Am J Clin Oncol 11 [Suppl 2]:S152–S155

Combination Therapy with Flutamide and Castration (Orchiectomy or LH-RH Agonist) in Untreated Patients with Advanced Prostate Cancer

A. Dupont, F. Labrie, L. Cusan, J. L. Gomez, M. Tremblay, Y. Lacourcière, J. Emond, and G. Monfette

Medical Research Council Group in Molecular Endocrinology, CHUL Research Center and Laval University, Quebec GIV 4G2, Canada

Introduction

Since the observations reported by Huggins and his colleagues (1941), the standard treatment of advanced prostate cancer has been a choice between orchiectomy and estrogens (Huggins and Hodges 1941; Nesbit and Baum 1950; Jordan et al. 1977; Mettlin et al. 1982; Murphy et al. 1983). Following such neutralization of testicular androgens, a positive response is observed in 60% – 80% of patients for a limited time interval, thus leaving 20% – 40% of patients in progression without any effect of treatment. Moreover, in the 60% – 80% of patients who initially respond, relapse of the disease is usually seen within 6 – 24 months (Resnick and Grayhack 1975) and 50% of them are expected to die within the next 5 months (Johnson et al. 1977; Slack and Murphy 1984).

A recent endocrine finding of major importance in this field is the discovery that androgens of adrenal origin play a role of almost equal importance to that of testicular androgens in prostate cancer (for reviews, see Labrie et al. (1988 a) and Labrie (1991). In addition to convincing biochemical evidence (Labrie et al. 1985, 1988 a), the unequivocal role of adrenal androgens in the growth of human prostate cancer after castration is clearly demonstrated by the numerous studies showing a 30% – 50% objective response to hypophysectomy, aminoglutethimide, or adrenalectomy in patients in relapse after orchiectomy or estrogen treatment (Labrie et al. 1985; Murray and Pitt 1985; Maddy et al. 1971; Labrie et al. 1986).

Since the development of tumor heterogeneity as well as resistance to treatment is likely to result from a treatment limited to the partial blockade of androgens (Labrie et al. 1985; Labrie and Veilleux 1986), and since flutamide, a well-tolerated and pure antiandrogen devoid of any other antihormonal or hormonal activity (Neri et al. 1972; Poyet and Labrie 1985), is available, we have used a combination therapy of flutamide and castration (surgical or luteinizing hormone releasing hormone, LH-RH, agonist) in 262 patients presenting with clinical stage D2 prostate cancer without previous endocrine therapy.

Recent Results in Cancer Research, Vol. 124
© Springer-Verlag Berlin · Heidelberg 1992

It is well recognized that a major problem facing the treatment of advanced prostate cancer is the choice of therapy in the 20%–40% of patients who do not respond to orchiectomy, estrogens, or LH-RH agonists alone. The same problem arises after some delay for all the remaining 60%–80% of patients who initially responded, but then usually showed progression of their cancer within 6–24 months (Resnick and Grayhack 1975). For those patients, the median life expectancy from the time of progression is then limited to approximately 6 months (Johnson et al. 1977; Slack and Murphy 1984).

In fact, much of the clinical evidence which has accumulated since the first adrenalectomy was performed by Huggins in 1945 (Huggins and Scott 1945) clearly shows that androgen-sensitive prostatic tumors remain after castration (surgical or medical), since the growth of these tumors is stimulated by androgens of adrenal origin. As mentioned above, these data pertain to the observation that further androgen blockade achieved by hypophysectomy, adrenalectomy, or aminoglutethimide in patients showing relapse induces a positive response in a large proportion of them (Labrie et al. 1985; Murray and Pitt 1985; Maddy et al. 1971). Since the aim of all these therapies is to block the secretion and/or action of adrenal androgens, a logical approach appears to be the use of a pure antiandrogen, such as flutamide, a drug which has a high specific action limited to the blockade of the androgen receptor in target tissues such as the prostate.

Patients and Methods

Starting in 1982, 262 patients with histologically proven prostate adenocarcinoma and distant metastases (stage D2) took part in our study after written consent. The mean duration of treatment was 1087 days (range 26–3154). The criteria for inclusion and exclusion were those of the United States National Prostate Cancer Project (NPCP) (Slack and Murphy 1984; Labrie et al. 1988 b), except that a short life expectancy was not used as criteria for exclusion. All patients presenting with stage D2 prostate cancer and who had received no previous endocrine therapy or chemotherapy were thus included, the only exclusions being patients with a second cancer. The patients with very advanced disease and a short life expectancy were not excluded in order to more closely mimic the situation found in usual urological practice. Demographic data and baseline profiles for patients who received the combination therapy are shown in Table 1. In this study, pain and abnormal performance were found in 161 (61.4%) and 96 (36.6%) patients, respectively. Sixty-one patients had diffused and disseminated bone metastases, while a mean of nine lesions per subject was calculated for the remaining patients.

The LH-RH agonist was injected subcutaneously at a daily dose of 500 µg at 0800 hours for 1 month followed by a 250 µg daily dose, while 250 mg flutamide was given orally three times daily at 0700, 1500, and 2300 hours. The antiandrogen was started 2 h or 1 day before the first administration of the LH-RH agonist or orchiectomy as described by Labrie et al. (1990). Complete

Table 1. Demographic data and baseline profiles for patients study using combination of LH-RH agonist, orchiectomy, and flutamide therapy

Number	262
Mean age in years (range)	66 (38–86)
ECOG performance status	
0–2	90
3–4	6
Bone pain	161
Pathologic fractures	2
Severe disease	60
Regional nodal involvement	37
Distant nodal involvement	44
Lung or pleural involvement	5
Liver involvement	1
Metastatic bone involvement	
Pelvic involvement	70
Rib involvement	69
Vertebral involvement	76
Long bone involvement	34
Skull involvement	21
Elevated acid phosphatase	229

ECOG, Eastern Cooperative Oncology Group.

clinical, urological, biochemical and radiological evaluation of the patients was performed before starting treatment as described previously (Labrie et al. 1983, 1985).

Since the results obtained using the same criteria in all the recent studies on the blockade of testicular androgens achieved by various approaches have yielded almost superimposable results (Murphy et al. 1983; Smith et al. 1985; Leuprolide Study Group 1984; Raynaud 1988; Béland et al. 1988; Crawford et al. 1989), thus indicating the reliability of the criteria used, we have compared the present results with those obtained in those recent studies performed with comparable populations of patients at the same stage of the disease.

Results

As illustrated in Fig. 1, a positive objective response assessed according to the criteria of the United States NPCP (Slack and Murphy 1984) was obtained in 234 of 257 patients (93.2%), thus leaving only 17 patients (6.8%) with no response to the treatment. The most striking effect is seen on complete responses, which have been observed in 30.3% of patients as compared with an average of only 4.6% in the five recent studies limited to a blockade of testicular androgens (Murphy et al. 1983; Smith et al. 1985; Leuprolide Study Group 1984). The rate of complete objective response is thus increased by more than six fold ($p < 0.01$; Fig. 1). The other striking finding illustrated in Fig. 1 is that only 6.8% of patients did not show an objective response at the

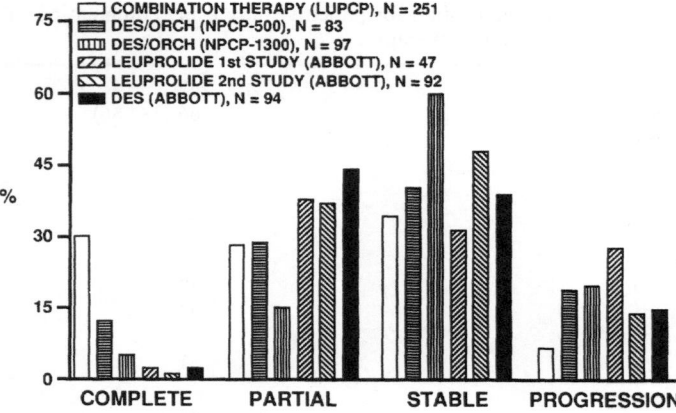

Fig. 1. Comparison of the best objective response rates (complete and partial response stable condition, and disease progression) assessed according to the United States NPCP criteria following combination therapy with flutamide (*LUPCP,* Laval University Prostate Cancer Program) and the five comparable studies using orchiectomy, DES, or leuprolide alone. (Murphy et al. 1983; Smith et al. 1985; Leuprolide Study Group 1984)

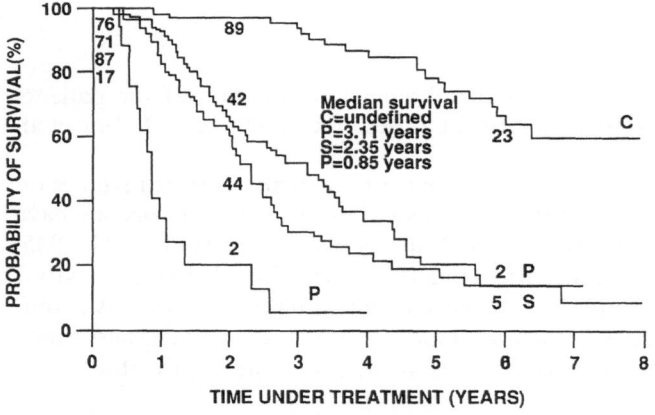

Fig. 2. Probability of survival according to the best objective response achieved (*c,* complete; *p,* partial; *s,* stable; or *p,* disease progression) following combination therapy

start of the combination therapy, while an average of 18% of patients continued to progress upon initiation of monotherapy (orchiectomy, diethylstilbestrol, DES, or leuprolide alone) in the other studies, thus representing an almost threefold difference ($p < 0.01$).

It is of interest to see in Fig. 2 that the classification of patients according to the four categories of responses of the United States NPCP has major prognostic value. The group of 17 nonresponders has an average 50% life expectancy of only 0.85 years compared with those who had a partial or stable response who display a median survival time of 3.11 and 2.35 years, respective-

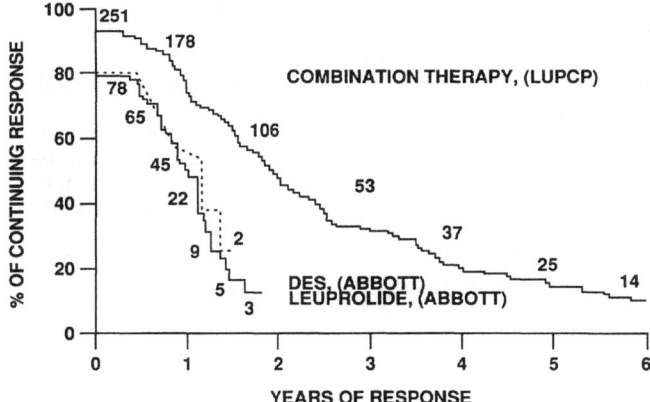

Fig. 3. Comparison of the probability of continuing response following combination therapy and the administration of leuprolide alone or DES (Leuprolide Study Group, 1984). The numbers on the curve correspond to the number of patients at risk at each indicated time interval

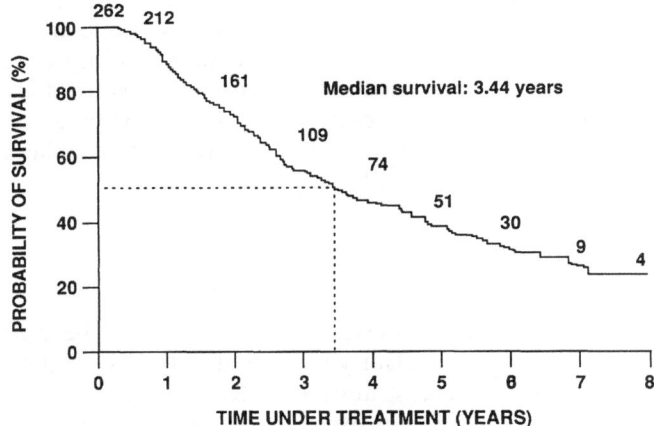

Fig. 4. Probability of survival following combination therapy. *Dotted line* indicates the median survival. The numbers on the curve correspond to the number of patients at risk at each indicated time interval

ly; however, the best probability of survival is seen in those who achieved a complete response, and the median survival has still not been reached after 8 years. Figure 3 illustrates the probability of continuing response. The median duration of response is 2.23 years. The probability of continuing response is 82% at 1 year (179 patients), 55% at 2 years (106 patients), 39% at 3 years (63 patients), 28% at 4 years (37 patients), and 22% at 5 years (25 patients). The median survival time was estimated at 3.44 years, the probability of survival at 1, 2, 3, 4, 5, 6, 7, and 8 years being 88.5%, 71.7%, 55.2%, 45.8%, 38.1%, 31.0%, 26.1%, and 23.2%, respectively (Fig. 4). Comparison of the survival

Table 2. Comparison of median survival times observed in the most recent studies using combination therapy and monotherapy

Studies	Disease-free survival (months)		Survival (months)	
	LH-RH agonist/ orchiectomy	Combi- nation therapy	LH-RH agonist/ orchiectomy	Combi- nation therapy
Crawford et al. (1989)	13.9	16.5	28.3	35.6
Anandron study (Raynaud, 1988, Béland et al., 1988)	12	17	19	33
LUPCP[a] (present study)		26.7		41.3
Leuprolide study (The Leuprolide Study Group, 1984)	13.8		Not estimated	
NPCP-500 (Murphy et al., 1983)	11.6		21.6	

[a] LUPCP, Laval University Prostate Cancer Program.

times observed following combination therapy and those recently obtained with DES, orchiectomy, or LH-RH agonist alone are illustrated in Table 2.

Performance status was rapidly and markedly improved. Ninety-six patients (36.6%) had an abnormal performance at the start of treatment as compared with only five patients 6 months later. In the 161 patients who had pain before starting combination therapy, only 12 were still complaining of pain related to their cancer after 6 months.

Discussion

The present data obtained in this study using the objective criteria of the United States NPCP clearly indicate that the use of the combination therapy with flutamide and castration (LH-RH agonist or orchiectomy) significantly increases the rate of objective response, the duration of response, and survival compared with monotherapies (orchiectomy, DES, or leuprolide alone) in previously untreated patients with clinical stage D2 prostate cancer.

It is well recognized that a positive correlation is observed between the incidence of the objective responses and survival (Labrie et al. 1988; Murphy et al. 1983). In fact, the patients who achieve a complete objective response have the best prognosis, while those who achieve partial or stable response as best response have a shorter life expectancy. On the other hand, the patients who show no response to treatment have a poor prognosis, with a median life expectancy of only 10 months. As previously shown in study 500 of the United States NPCP and confirmed in the present study (Fig. 2), patients who show a complete response have a better probability of survival. In fact, it is well known that patients who do not respond to endocrine therapy or continue to progress at the start of treatment have an extremely poor prognosis, the median life expectancy being approximately 6 months (Johnson et al. 1977). The decreased percentage of nonresponders from 18% to 6.8% clearly illustrates the inhibitory effect of combination therapy on adrenal steroids. Since the rate of partial and stable response is not appreciably different between monotherapy and dual combination therapy, the major difference observed between standard therapy and combination therapy is a shift of patients from the category of non-responders (short life expectancy and poor quality of life) into that of complete responders (increased life expectancy and good quality of life).

When compared with recent data obtained with monotherapies, the present study shows that combination therapy causes a 5.3-fold increase in the number of patients who achieved a complete response (from 4.8% to 30.3%) while the percentage of nonresponders decreased from 18% to 6.8%. Thus, as early as in 1950, Nesbit and Baum (1950) reported an avarage survival of 9.6 months after the onset of relapse in 213 patients who received estrogen upon relapse after orchiectomy, and vice versa. In a series of 327 patients showing relapse after castration, 50% were dead at 7 months after first evidence of relapse (Brendler and Prout 1962; Brendler 1969). In addition to providing an improvement in the quality of life, the observed increase in the number of complete responses and a decrease in the proportion of non-responders leads to 1.5 years of additional survival. In the Intergroup study, the combination of complete and partial responders was 43% for combination therapy compared with 35% for monotherapy (Crawford et al. 1989). Similarly, in the Anandron study, 46% of patients achieved complete or partial responses in the orchiectomy plus Anandron group, while the same best response was obtained in only 20% of patients treated with orchiectomy and placebo (Béland et al. 1988). In the same study, 38% of patients did not respond to orchiectomy alone, while the percentage of nonresponders decreased to 20% following combination therapy. In fact, all the randomized trials comparing medical or surgical castration in association with a pure antiandrogen (flutamide or Anandron) with castration, and analyzed after a sufficiently long time, have shown the advantages of the combination therapy on: the best response achieved; the duration of response; and, even more importantly, on survival (Crawford et al. 1989; Raynaud 1988; Béland et al. 1988). Since the advantages of the antiandrogen have been observed in combination with both orchiectomy (Raynaud 1988; Béland et al. 1988; Brisset et al. 1987; Namer et al. 1988) and LH-RH agonists (Navratil 1987; Crawford et al. 1989; and this study), the benefits are not limited to prevention of flare of the disease during the first days of treatment with an LH-RH agonist, but are secondary to the inhibition of the antiandrogen of the action of the adrenal androgens.

It is well recognized that the "apparently low" levels of plasma testosterone (T) and dihydrotestosterone (DHT) remaining after surgical or medical castration in men do not properly reflect the degree of inhibition of androgen action in target tissues (Labrie et al. 1985; Geller et al. 1988). The main androgen precursors of adrenal origin in men are dehydroepiandrosterone (DHEA) (25 mg/day) and androstenedione (Δ^4-dione) 3 mg/day (Sanford et al. 1977).

Man is unique among animals species in having adrenals that secrete large amounts of the inactive precursor steroids DHEA and especially its sulfate (DHEA-S) which are converted into potent androgens in peripheral tissues. Adrenal secretion of DHEA and DHEA-S increases during the adrenarche in children at the age of 6–8 years and very high values of circulating DHEA-S are maintained through adulthood (Labrie et al. 1985; de Peretti and Forest 1978; Cutler et al. 1978; Adams 1985; Brochu and Bélanger 1987). In fact, plasma DHEA-S levels in adult men are 100–500 times higher than those of testosterone.

The first bilateral adrenalectomy in prostate cancer was performed by Huggins and Scott (1945) with appreciable success despite the lack of substitution therapy. Subsequently, bilateral adrenalectomy was used in advanced prostate cancer with a significant rate of remission in previously castrated patients or those already treated with estrogens. Bilateral adrenalectomy has been found to be associated with palliation in 20%–70% of patients with advanced prostate carcinoma who had become refractory to castration or estrogen therapy (Bhanalaph et al. 1974; Sanford et al. 1977; Ferguson 1975; MacFarlane et al. 1960; Morales et al. 1955; Harrison et al. 1953). A similar rate of response has been observed with medical adrenalectomy using aminoglutethimide (Robinson et al. 1974; Ponder et al. 1984; Drago et al. 1984; Worgul et al. 1983).

This situation of a high secretion rate of precursor adrenal androgens in men is thus completely different from all animal models used in the laboratory, namely rats, mice, guinea pigs, monkeys, or others, where the secretion of sex steroids takes place exclusively in the gonads (Labrie et al. 1985; Bélanger et al. 1989 and refs therein). These findings open a new field of endocrinology, namely that of intracrine secretion. Through intracrine activity, locally produced androgens and/or estrogens exert their action inside the same cells where synthesis takes place. The term "intracrine activity" has been recently introduced as this new section of endocrinology (Labrie et al. 1988), a terminology complementary to the well-known autocrine, paracrine, and endocrine activities where a hormone is active at the surface of the producing cells (autocrine), a hormone is acting on neighboring cells (paracrine) or a hormone released in the circulation is acting on distant target tissues (endocrine).

The most direct and straightforward evidence of an important role for adrenal androgens in prostate cancer is the finding that the active androgen DHT remains at physiologically active concentrations in prostate cancer tissue following removal of testis androgens by orchiectomy or treatment with estrogens or LH-RH agonists. In fact, a high concentration of the active androgen DHT remains in prostate cancer tissue following castration. Although orchiectomy, estrogens, or LH-RH agonists (through blockade of release of bioactive LH) cause a 90%–95% reduction in serum testosterone (T) concentration (Warner et al. 1973; Labrie et al. 1980; Waxman et al. 1983; Labrie et al. 1985), a much smaller effect is observed on the only meaningful parameter of androgenic action, namely the concentration of DHT in prostate cancer tissue (Geller et al. 1988).

Measurements of T and DHT concentrations in serum have little or no value except as an index of testis activity. In fact, intraprostatic DHT concentration is the only significant parameter which indicates the level of androgenic activity at its site of action in prostatic cancer tissue.

As another measure of the importance of adrenal androgens in adult men, the serum levels of the main metabolites of androgens, namely 5α-androstane-3α,17β-diol (3α-diol), androsterone (ADT), and their glucuronidated derivatives, are only reduced by 50%–70% (Moghissi et al. 1984; Bélanger et al. 1986), thus reflecting the high level of adrenal precursors converted into DHT in castrated men.

It is now well demonstrated that the human prostate possesses all the enzymes required for the synthesis of active androgens from inactive adrenal steroid precursors, thus providing the explanation for the findings of intraprostatic concentrations of DHT as high as 1.5 ng/g tissue (4.5 nM) following surgical or medical castration (Labrie et al. 1988 b). With regard to the latter steroid, it might be relevant to recall that treatment with flutamide (250 mg, every 8 h) decreases intraprostatic DHT levels below 0.2 ng/g trissue (Labrie et al. 1987 a). Such findings are indicative of the efficiency of flutamide in displacing intraprostatic DHT from its intracellular receptor. Knowing that the K_d value of DHT interaction with the androgen receptor is less than 1 nM (Simard et al. 1986; Asselin et al. 1982), it is clear that a concentration of 1.5 nM DHT left in the prostate cancer tissue after castration will exert a major stimulatory effect on cancer growth.

In addition to the long-term beneficial effects of combination therapy, the use of flutamide at the start of treatment eliminates the unnecessary risks of disease flare which are known to occur in a significant proportion of patients treated with an LH-RH agonist alone (Labrie et al. 1987a; Waxman et al. 1983; Kahan et al. 1984; Labrie et al. 1984). With the undisputable knowledge that the adrenals contribute 30%–50% of total androgens in men, and with the positive results obtained in all studies using a pure antiandrogen (flutamide or Anandron) in association with medical or surgical castration, it seems logical to suggest that combination therapy should be the standard treatment for all patients suffering from advanced prostate cancer. Recently, the Medical Letter on Drugs and Therapeutics make the combination therapy of LH-RH analog plus flutamide the drugs of choice for treating prostate cancer.

References

Adams JB (1985) Control of secretion and the function of C19-delta-5-steroids of the human adrenal gland. Molec cell Endocr 45:1–17

Aseelin J, Mélançon R, Moachon G, Bélanger A (1980) Characteristics of binding to estrogen, androgen, progestin and glucocorticoid receptors in 7,12-dimethylbenz(a)anthracene-induced mammary tumors and their hormonal control. Cancer Res 40:1612–1622

Béland G, Elhilalı M, Fradet Y, Laroche B, Ramsey EW, Trachtenberg J, Venner PM, Tewari HD (1988) Total androgen blockade versus castration in metastatic cancer of the prostate. In: Motta M, Serio M (eds), Hormonal Therapy of Prostatic Diseases: Basic and Clincal Aspects, Medicom, Bussum pp 302–311

Bélanger A, Dupont A, Labrie F (1984) Inhibition of basal and adrenocorticotropin-stimulated plasma levels of adrenal androgens after treatment with an antiandrogen in castrated patients with prostatic cancer. J Clin Endocrinol Metab 59:422–426

Bélanger A, Brochu M, Cliche J (1986) Levels of plasma steroid glucuronides in intact and castrated men with prostatic cancer. J Clin Endocrinol Metab 62:812–815

Bélanger B, Bélanger A, Labrie F, Dupont A, Cusan L, Monfette G (1989) Comparison of residual C-19 steroids in plasm and prostatic tissue of human, rat and guinea pig after castration: unique importance of extratesticular androgen in men. J Steroid Biochem 32:695–698

Bhanalaph T, Varkarakis MJ, Murphy GP (1974) Current status of bilateral adrenalectomy of advanced prostatic cancer. J Clin Endocrinol Metab 59:422–426

Brendler H (1969) Current cancer concepts: therapy with orchiectomy or estrogens or both. JAMA 210:1074–1075

Brendler H, Prout GR Jr (1962) A cooperative group study of prostatic cancer. Stilbestrol versus placebo in advanced progressive disease. Cancer Chemother Rep 16:323–327

Brisset JM, Bertagna C, Fiet K, de Gery A, Hucher M, Husson JM, Tremblay D, Raynaud JP (1987) Total androgen blockade versus orchiectomy in stage D prostate cancer. In: Klijn JGM (ed) Hormonal Manipulation of Cancer: Peptides Growth Factors and New (anti)steroidal agents, vol 18, Raven Press, New York, pp 17–30

Brochu M, Bélanger A (1987) Increase in plasma steroid glucuronide levels in men from infancy to adulthood. J Cell Endocr Metab 64:1283–1287

Crawford ED, Eisenberger MA, McLeod DG, Spaulding JT, Benson R, Door FA, Blumenstein DA, Davis MA, Goodman PJ (1989) A controlled trial of leuprolide with and without Flutamide in prostatic carcinoma. New Engl J Med 321:419–424

Cutler GB Jr, Glenn M, Bush M, Hodgen GD, Graham CE, Loriaux DL (1978) Adrenarche: a survey of rodents, domestic animals and primates. Endocrinology 103:2112–2118

de Peretti E, de Forest MG (1978) Pattern of plasma dehydroepiandrosterone sulfate levels in human from birth to adulthood. Evidence for testicular production. J Cell Endocr Metab 47:572–577

Drago JR, Santen RJ, Lipton A, Worgul TJ, Harvey HA, Boucher A, Manni A, Rohner TJ (1984) Clinical effect of aminoglutethimide, medical adrenalectomy in treatment of 43 patients with advanced prostatic carcinoma. Cancer 53:1447–1450

Ferguson JD (1975) Limits and indication for adrenalectomy and hypophysectomy in the treatment of prostatic cancer. In: Bracci U, Di Silverio F (eds) Hormonal Therapy of Prostatic Cancer, Cofese Edizioni, Palermo, pp 201–207

Geller J, Albert J, Nachtseim DA, Loza DC (1988) Advantages of total androgen blockade in the treatment of advanced prostate cancer. Semin Oncol 15:53–61

Harper ME, Pike A, Peeling WB, Griffiths K (1974) Steroids of adrenal origin metabolized by human prostatic tissue both in vivo and in vitro. J Endocr 60:117–125

Harrison JH, Thorn GW, Jenkins D (1953) Total adrenalectomy for reactivated carcinoma of the prostate. N Engl J Med 248:86–92

Huggins C, Hodges CV (1941) Studies of prostatic cancer. I. Effect of castration, estrogen and androgen injections on serum phosphatases in metastatic carcinoma of the prostate. Cancer Res 1:293–297

Huggins C, Scott WW (1945) Bilateral adrenalectomy in prostatic cancer. Ann Surg 122:1031

Johnson DE, Scott WW, Gibbons RP, Prout GR, Schmidt JD, Chu JTM, Gaeta J, Sarott J, Murphy GP (1977) National randomized study of chemotherapeutic agents in advanced prostatic carcinoma: progress report. Cancer Treat Rep 61:317–323

Jordan WP Jr, Blackard CE, Byar DP (1977) Reconsideration of orchiectomy in the treatment of advanced prostatic carcinoma. S Afr Med J 70:1411–1413

Kahan A, Delrieu F, Amor B, Chiche R, Steg A (1984) Disease flare induced by D-Trp[6]-GnRH analogue in patients with metastatic prostatic cancer. Lancet 1:971–972

Labrie C, Bélanger A, Labrie F (1988) Androgenic activity of dehydroepiandrosterone and androstenedione in the rat ventral prostate. Endocrinology 123:1412–1417

Labrie F, Veilleux R (1986) A wide range of sensitivities to androgens develops in cloned Shionogi mouse mammary tumor cells. Prostate 8:293–300

Labrie F, Dupont A, Bélanger A, Lacourcière Y, Raynaud JP, Husson JM, Gareau J, Fazekas ATA, Sandow J, Monfette G, Girard JG, Emond J, Houle JG (1983) New approach in the treatment of prostate cancer: complete instead of only partial withdrawal of androgens. Prostate 4:579–594

Labrie F, Dupont A, Bélanger A, Emond J, Monfette G (1984) Simultaneous administration of pure antiandrogens, a combination necessary for the use of luteinizing hormone-releasing hormone agonists in the treatment of prostate cancer. Proc Nat Acad Sci U.S.A. 81:3861–3863

Labrie F, Dupont A, Bélanger A (1985) Complete androgen blockade for the treatment of prostate cancer. In: De Vita VT, Hellman S, Rosenberg SA (eds) Important Advances in Oncology, Lippincott, Philadelphia, pp 193–217

Labrie F, Dupont A, Bélanger A, St-Arnaud R, Giguère M, Lacourciere Y, Emond J, Monfette G (1986) Treatment of prostate cancer with gonadotropin-releasing hormone agonists. Endocr Rev 7:67–74

Labrie F, Dupont A, Bélanger A, Lachance R (1987a) Flutamide eliminates the risk of disease flare in prostate cancer patients treated with an LHRH agonist. J Urol 138:804–806

Labrie F, Luthy L, Veilleux R, Simard J, Bélanger A, Dupont A (1987b) New concepts on the androgen sensitivity of prostate cancer. In Murphy G (ed) Proc 2nd Int Symp on Prostate Cancer, Alan Liss, New York, pp 145–72

Labrie F, Bélanger A, Veilleux R, Lacoste D, Labrie C, Marchetti B, Poulin R, Dupont A, Cusan L, Luthy I (1988a) Rationale for maximal androgen withdrawal in the therapy of prostate cancer. Baillière's Clin Oncol 2:597–619

Labrie F, Dupont A, Giguère M, Cusan L, Bergeron N, Emond J, Monfette G, Lacourcière Y, Boucher H, Lachance R (1988b) Important prognostic value of standardized objective criteria of response in stage D2 prostatic carcinoma. Eur J Cancer Clin Oncol 12:1869–1878

Labrie F, Dupont A, Cusan L, Gomez JL, Emond J, Monfette G (1990) Combination therapy with flutamide and medical (LHRH agonist) or surgical castration in advanced prostate cancer: 7-year clinical experience. J Steroid Biochem 37:943–950

Labrie F (1991) Treatment of prostate cancer. In: Strauss III, JF (ed) Endocrinology and Metabolism Clinics of North America, W. B. Saunders, in press

Leuprolide Study Group (1984) Leuprolide versus diethylstilbestrol for metastatic prostate cancer. N Engl J Med 311:1281–1286

MacFarlane DA, Thomas LP, Harrison JH (1960) A survey of total adrenalectomy in cancer of the prostate. Am J Surg 99:562–572

Maddy JA, Winternitz WW, Norrell H (1971) Cryohypophysectomy in the management of advanced prostatic cancer. Cancer 28:322–328

Medical Letter (1991) Drugs of choice for cancer chemotherapy. The Medical Letter on Drugs and Therapeutics 33 (issue 840, March 22)

Mettlin C, Natarajan N, Murphy GP (1982) Recent patterns of care of prostatic cancer patients in the United States: results from the surveys of the American College of Surgeons Commission on Cancer. Int Adv Surg Oncol 5:277–321

Moghissi E, Alban F, Horton R (1984) Origin of plasma androstanediol glucuronide in men. J Clin Endocrinol Metab 59:417–421

Morales PA, Brendler H, Hotchkiss RS (1955) The role of the adrenal cortex in prostatic cancer. J Urol 73:399–409

Murphy GP, Beckley S, Brady MF, Chu M, DeKernion JB, Dhabuwala C, Gaeta JF, Gibbons RP, Loening S, McKieri CF, McLeod DG, Pontes JE, Prout GR, Scardino PT,

Schlegel JU, Schmidt JD, Scott WW, Slack NH, Soloway M (1983) Treatment of newly diagnosed metastatic prostate cancer patients with chemotherapy agents in combination with hormones versus hormones alone. Cancer 51:1264–1272

Murray R, Pitt P (1985) Treatment of advanced prostatic cancer resistant to conventional therapy with aminoglutethimide. Eur J Cancer Clin Oncol 21:453–458

Namer M, Amiel J, Toubol J (1988) Anandron (RU23908) associated with orchiectomy in stage D prostate cancer: preliminary results of a randomized double-blind study. Am J Clin Oncol 11 (Suppl 2):S191–S196

Narayana AS, Loening SA, Culp DA (1981) Flutamide in the treatment of metastatic carcinoma of the prostate. Br J Urol 52:152–153

Navratil H (1987) Double-blind study of Anandron versus placebo in stage D2 prostate cancer patients receiving buserelin. Progress Clin Biol Res 243A:401–410

Neri R, Florance K, Koziol P, Van Cleave S (1972) A biological profile of a non-steroidal antiandrogen, SCH13521 (4'-nitro-3'-trifluoromethylisobutyranilide). Endocrinology 91:427–437

Nesbit RM, Baum WC (1950) Endocrine control of prostatic carcinoma: clinical and statistical survey of 1818 cases. JAMA 143:1317–1320

Ponder BAJ; Shearer RJ, Pocock RD, Miller J, Easton D, Chilvers CED, Dowsett M, Jeffcoate SL (1984) Response to aminoglutethimide and cortisone acetate in advanced prostatic cancer. Br J Cancer 50:757–763

Poyet P, Labrie F (1985) Comparison of the antiandrogenic/androgenic activities of flutamide, cyproterone acetate and megestrol acetate. Mol Cell Endocrinol 42:283–288

Raynaud JP (1988) Antiandrogens in combination with LHRH agonist in prostate cancer. Am J Clin Oncol 11 (Suppl 2):S132–S147

Resnick MI, Grayhack JT (1975) Treatment of stage IV carcinoma of the prostate. Urol Clin North Am 2:141–161

Robinson MRG, Shearer RJ, Fergusson JD (1974) Adrenal suppression in the treatment of carcinoma of the prostate. Br J Urol 46:555–559

Sanford EJ, Paulson DF, Rohner TJ, Drago JR, Santen RJ, Bardin CW (1977) The effects of castration on adrenal testosterone secretion in men with prostatic carcinoma. J Urol 118:1019–1021

Simard J, Luthy I, Guay J, Bélanger A, Labrie F (1986) Characteristics of interaction of the antiandrogen Flutamide with the androgen receptor in various target tissues. Mol Cell Endocrinol 8:293–300

Slack NH, Murphy GD (1984) NPCP Participants: criteria for evaluating patient responses to treatment modalities for prostatic cancer. Urol Clin North Am 11:337–342

Smith JA, Glode LM, Wettlaufer JN, Strein BS, Glass AG, Max DT, Anbar D, Jagst CL, Murphy G (1985) Clinical effects of gonadotropin-releasing hormone analogue in metastatic carcinoma of the prostate. Urology 20:106–114

Sogani PC, Ray B, Whitmore WF Jr (1975) Advanced prostatic carcinoma: flutamide therapy after conventional endocrine treatment. Urology 6:164–166

Stoliar B, Albert DJ (1974) SCH 1352 in the treatment of advanced carcinoma of the prostate. J Urol 111:803–807

Warner B, Worgul TJ, Drago J, Demers L, Dufau M. Max D, Santen RJ, Abbott Study Group (1973) Effect of very high doses of D-leucine-6-gonadotropin-releasing hormone proethylamide on the hypothalamic-pituitary testicular axis in patients with prostatic cancer. J Clin Invest 71:1842–1855

Waxman JH, Was JAH, Hendry WF, Whitfield HN, Besser GM, Malpas JS, Olivier RTD (1983) Treatment with gonadotropin-releasing hormone analogue in advanced prostatic cancer. Brit Med J 286:1309–1312

Worgul TJ, Santen RJ, Samojlik E, Veldhuis JD, Lipton A, Harvey HA, Drago JR, Rohner TJ (1983) Clinical and biochemical effect of aminoglutethimide in the treatment of advanced prostatic carcinoma. J Urol 129:51–55

LH-RH Agonists in the Treatment of Ovarian Cancer

G. Emons[1,2], O. Ortmann[1,2], G. S. Pahwa[2], F. Oberheuser[2], and K.-D. Schulz[1]

[1] Zentrum für Frauenheilkunde und Geburtshilfe, Philipps-Universität Marburg, Pilgrimstein 3, W-3550 Marburg, FRG
[2] Klinik für Frauenheilkunde und Geburtshilfe, Medizinische Universität Lübeck, Ratzeburger Allee 160, W-2400 Lübeck, FRG

Introduction

Ovarian carcinoma is one of the most common causes of cancer death in women. During the last decade there have been some advances in surgical, radiation, and cytotoxic chemotherapy of this malignancy. The overall results of these treatments, however, are still disappointing (MRC Gynecologic Cancer Working Party 1990; Averette and Donato 1990; Blackledge and Lawton 1989). Aggressive chemotherapy is burdened with severe acute side effects. In addition, chemotherapy in ovarian cancer is associated with a 4–12 times higher risk of developing leukemia (Kaldor et al. 1990). One trend in modern oncology has been to reduce at least therapy-induced morbidity, if the efficacy of therapy cannot be improved by increased aggressiveness. With breast and endometrial cancer this has been successfully achieved by the introduction of endocrine treatments, both ablative or additive, that take advantage of the sex-steroid dependence of some of these tumors, as reflected by the presence of estrogen and/or progestin receptors (Desombre et al. 1987). Also many ovarian cancers contain significant amounts of sex-steroid receptors. Therapeutic approaches, however, using either antiestrogens or progestins, have not been satisfying (for review, see Desombre et al. 1987; Rao and Slotman 1991).

It has been known for over one hundred years that married women are much less prone to develop ovarian cancer than unmarried women (Olshausen 1877). Some authors believed that this phenomenon was due to the suppression of the libido in unmarried women, which caused hyperemia of the genital organs. The majority of gynecologists at that time supposed however, that the higher incidence of ovarian cancer in unmarried women was caused by menstrual hyperemia, which occurred naturally more often in this population than in married women, who menstruated less due to pregnancies, childbed, and lactation (for review, see Mayer 1925). Since the 1970s it has been shown by many investigators that the number of pregnancies and the duration of the use of oral contraceptives are significantly inversely related to the incidence of ovarian cancer (Fathalla 1971; Casagrande et al. 1979; Kvale et al. 1988; Schlesselman 1989). Fathalla (1971) first suggested that the incessant monthly ovulation which is typical for our species, at least in the twentieth century, is a causal factor for the development of ovarian cancer since the coelomic epithelium is repeatedly ruptured. Other authors (e.g., Stadel 1975; Cramer and Welch 1983) suggested that exposure to the relevant gonadotropin levels in cycling women might favor the development of ovarian cancer. This "gonadotropin theory" is further supported by the steep increase of the incidence of ovarian carcinoma with the advent of the menopause, when gonadotropin levels rise physiologically (e.g., Stadel 1975; Schlesselman 1989). If ovarian cancer was luteinizing hormone (LH)- and/or follicle-stimulating hormone (FSH)-dependent, suppression of gonadotropins, which is nowadays most effectively achieved with luteinizing hormone releasing hormone (LH-RH) analogs, should be beneficial for patients suffering from this disease.

During the past few years, a number of groups have reported on the direct effects of LH-RH analogs on several human extrapituitary tissues, and an autocrine mechanism using LH-RH has been convincingly proposed for the human placenta. The synthesis of LH-RH (e.g., Siler-Khodr and Khodr 1980; Radovick et al. 1990), the presence of binding sites (e.g., Currie et al. 1981; Iwashita et al. 1986), and the biological activity of LH-RH in the human placenta (e.g., Belisle et al. 1984) could be demonstrated. This LH-RH autocrine system of the placenta seems to be integrated into other endocrine feedback systems (for review, see Petraglia et al. 1990).

A similar autocrine system based on LH-RH has been proposed for human breast cancer, and the in situ production of LH-RH could be demonstrated (e.g., Seppälä and Wahlström 1980; Bützow et al. 1987). The presence of specific binding sites for LH-RH in human breast cancer tissue and cell lines has been shown by different authors (e.g. Miller et al. 1985; Bützow et al. 1987; Eidne et al. 1987; Fekete et al. 1989 a). Direct effects of LH-RH analogs on breast cancer cell lines have now been established (Miller et al. 1985; Blankenstein et al. 1985; Scambia et al. 1988; Wilding et al. 1987; Mullen et al. 1991), although there had been some controversy on this subject. Levy and colleagues (1989) could show that in human breast cancer the classical LH-RH signal transduction mechanism can be activated by LH-RH analogs. An LH-RH-dependent autocrine system is also supposed in human prostate cancer (e.g., Qayum et al. 1990 a, b).

As early as 1982, Lamberts and coworkers (1982) showed that in a human ovarian tumor, an arrhenoblastoma, testosterone secretion could be directly inhibited by an LH-RH agonist. This finding has raised the question of whether an LH-RH-dependent autocrine mechanism which could be used for novel therapeutic approaches might also exist in human ovarian tumors, and especially in carcinomata.

Effects of LH-RH-Agonist-Induced Suppression of Gonadotropins on the Proliferation of Ovarian Cancer

In 1981, Rajaniemi et al. (1981) found LH (human chorionic gonadotropin) [LH(hCG)] receptors in 18% of benign human ovarian tumors and in 27% of malignant ones. Although the receptor content was low, their presence could be definitely shown in 6 out of 21 malignant epithelial tumors and in 1 out of 4 malignant granulosa cell tumors. In the same year, Kammerman et al. (1981) demonstrated hCG and FSH binding and gonadotropin-induced cyclic adenosine monophosphate (cAMP) production in some benign and malignant epithelial tumors as well as in sex-cord stromal and germ cell tumors.

These findings were disputed by Stouffer et al. (1984), who failed to find gonadotropin receptors in epithelial ovarian tumors. Only in a sex-cord stromal tumor did they find relevant FSH binding. Nakano et al. (1989) analyzed 29 ovarian tumors and found LH binding in one cystadenoma and in one theca cell tumor. Binding sites for FSH were found in three benign epithelial tumors and in two sex-cord stromal neoplasms. A surface-binding autoradiographic study described in the same paper showed that the binding sites for gonadotropins were localized in the stromal tissue. Recently, Ohtani (1990) analyzed 18 malignant ovarian tumors (17 of epithelial origin) and found specific FSH binding in 91%.

Simon and colleagues were able to stimulate DNA synthesis and proliferation in a number of ovarian cancer cell lines in vitro by hCG and FSH (Simon and Hölzel 1979; Simon et al. 1983). Hofmann and coworkers (1989) recently demonstrated that hCG preparations can be contaminated by epidermal growth factor (EGF)-related proteins. As EGF is a well-known mitogen for ovarian cancer cells (for review, see Bauknecht et al. 1988), care must be taken to discriminate between the actions of hCG and contaminating growth factors in tumor cell experiments. Ohtani (1990) tested 18 malignant ovarian tumors (17 of epithelial origin) in a subrenal capsule assay in the nude mouse. The xenograft size increased significantly under human menopausal gonadotropin (hMG) and human FSH (hFSH) treatment. This effect was most pronounced in patients that exhibited high FSH binding in vitro.

In a similar animal model, Peterson and Zimniski (1990) found that heterotransplanted human ovarian cancer (BG-1) had accelerated growth rates in surgically castrated nude mice with elevated gonadotropin levels as compared with intact controls.

Kullander et al. (1987) found that the growth of ovarian tumors in rats produced by autotransplantation of an ovary under the splenic capsule was inhibited by injections of the LH-RH agonist [D-Trp^6]-LH-RH. With the same LH-RH analog, Pour and coworkers (1989) decreased the growth of N-nitrosobis(2-oxopropyl)amine induced ovarian tumors in rats. Mortel et al. (1986) inhibited the growth of the human ovarian carcinoma cell line OVCAR-3 in nude mice with [D-Trp^6]-LH-RH. Also the results of Peterson and Zimniski (1990) favor the hypothesis that human ovarian cancer cell lines can grow gonadotropin-dependently in animals: as mentioned above, tumors from the

BG-1 human ovarian carcinoma line grew faster in castrated nude mice with elevated gonadotropin levels than in intact controls. When LH and FSH levels were suppressed below normal concentrations by injections of a long-acting LH-RH agonist (Lupron-SR), tumor growth rate was significantly reduced as compared with tumors in normal, intact animals, or in those treated with placebo.

These positive experimental results have encouraged a number of clinical pilot studies. In 1985 Parmar et al. (1985) reported on a patient with advanced ovarian cancer who relapsed after surgery, chemotherapy and radiotherapy, and who was then treated with [D-Trp[6]]-LH-RH. Concomitantly with the suppression of gonadotropins there was a marked shrinkage of the tumor masses. This partial remission lasted for 12 months. Later reports by Kullander et al. (1987), Parmar et al. (1988 a, b), Jäger et al. (1989), Kavanagh et al. (1989) and Bruckner and Motwani (1989) have shown that the reduction of LH and FSH levels achieved by the administration of LH-RH agonists can induce partial remission or lead to stable disease in 10% – 50% of patients with advanced ovarian cancer who have relapsed after conventional treatment. Kauppila and colleagues (1990) found beneficial effects of LH-RH agonist treatment in patients suffering from advanced ovarian granulosa cell malignancies. In this context a phase II study by Freedman et al. (1986) should be mentioned. A total of 65 patients with ovarian carcinoma that was refractory to chemotherapy were treated with a sequential regimen of ethynyl estradiol (50–100 µg/day) and medroxyprogesterone acetate (100–200 mg/day). Of these patients, 14% responded to treatment and 20% had stable disease. Although the interest of the authors was focused on direct steroid actions on the tumors, presumably mediated by progesterone receptors, the beneficial effects of their treatment might be also attributed to the suppression of gonadotropins that was probably achieved with the regimen used.

The experimental data and the results of the phase II clinical studies described above call for an evaluation in controlled clinical trials. Such a study is being performed at present by colleagues from Finland, Sweden, Israel and Germany (Fig. 1) (Emons et al. 1990). The trial is being carried out with patients, in whom an advanced ovarian cancer (Fédération Internationale de Gynecologie et Obstétrique, FIGO, stage III or IV) has been diagnosed for the first time. After surgical treatment and staging, the patients are randomized into groups, and receive either a long-acting preparation of [D-Trp[6]]-LH-RH (Decapeptyl, triptorelin, Depot) or placebo. For ethical reasons all patients

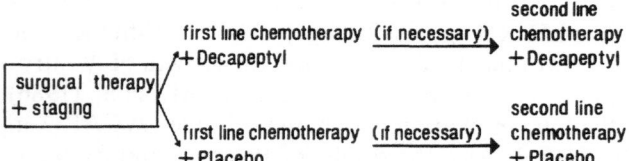

Fig. 1. Design of ovarian cancer study. (From Emons et al. 1990, with permission from Kluwer Academic Publishers)

receive a standardized first-line polychemotherapy (containing *cis*-platinum). Decapeptyl or placebo administration are additional and are continued if a second line chemotherapy is necessary. It will be accepted that the Decapeptyl therapy has an effect if survival times in the treatment group are at least 20% longer than in the control group. It is planned to recruit 200 patients. Up to now, approximately 90 women have entered the trial. In the patients treated with Decapeptyl, the suppression of gonadotropin levels is consistently observed. As to survival times, no statements can yet be made as observation times are still too short.

Direct Effects of LH-RH Analogs on Human Ovarian Carcinomata

In the rat, LH-RH has been described as a direct modulator of ovarian function. High-affinity, low-capacity receptors for LH-RH have been demonstrated in the ovaries of this species, comparable to pituitary LH-RH receptors (for review see Knecht et al. 1985; Hsueh and Schaeffer 1985). In the human ovary, comparable high-affinity, low-capacity LH-RH receptors were not found by Clayton and Huhtaniemi (1982). In later studies, low-affinity, high-capacity LH-RH binding sites have been characterized in human corpora lutea by Popkin et al. (1983) and Bramley et al. (1985) comparable to those in human placenta and breast cancer (see above).

Using a quantitative autoradiographic technique, Latouche et al. (1991) recently described high-affinity, low-capacity LH-RH receptors in human ovaries which were, however, exclusively localized on the granulosa cell layer of the dominant follicle. Li et al. (1987) characterized a gonadotropin-releasing peptide in human follicular fluid. Aten et al. (1987) described an LH-RH-like protein in human ovaries which might be part of an autocrine regulatory system.

As to direct effects of LH-RH on normal human ovarian tissue, the literature is controversial. Tureck et al. (1982) reported inhibition of human granulosa cell progesterone secretion by an LH-RH agonist. This finding has been contested by Casper et al. (1982). Also in human corpora lutea no direct LH-RH effects on progesterone production could be observed (Tan and Biggs 1983). Recently, Olsson and colleagues (1990) reported that an LH-RH agonist at relatively high concentrations exerted direct effects on gonadotropin-stimulated progesterone formation of human granulosa cells and that these effects were different (inhibitory or stimulatory) depending on the degree of follicular maturation. Pellicer and Miró (1990) found that the use of LH-RH agonists over a long period in in vitro fertilization cycles might affect the steroidogenic pathway of human granulosa luteal cells.

As a first step to elucidate possible direct effects of LH-RH analogs on ovarian cancer, our group checked whether or not LH-RH binding sites are present in these tumors. Using ^{125}I-labeled [D-Ala^6-desGly^{10}]-LH-RH ethyl-amide, we were able to demonstrate a low-affinity, high-capacity binding of this LH-RH agonist in plasma membranes from a number of human ovarian

Table 1. LH-RH binding sites in membranes from a selection of human ovarian carcinomata. (From Emons et al. 1989, with permission from Pergamon Press)

Material	Binding sites (10^{-12} M/mg protein)	K_a (10^5 M^{-1})
Highly differentiated serous cystadenocarcinoma	76	1.4
Poorly differentiated solid adenocarcinoma	16	2.3
Poorly differentiated serous carcinoma	212	0.8
Highly differentiated serous papillary adenocarcinoma	148	1.5
Poorly differentiated serous papillary adenocarcinoma	177	1.4
Poorly differentiated adenopapillary carcinoma	97	1.5
Highly differentiated serous papillary adenocarcinoma	301	1.7
Partly differentiated endometroid adenocarcinoma	330	1.0
Poorly differentiated adenocarcinoma	n.d.	n.d.
Partly differentiated, partly mucinous adenocarcinoma	n.d.	n.d.

n.d., not detected.

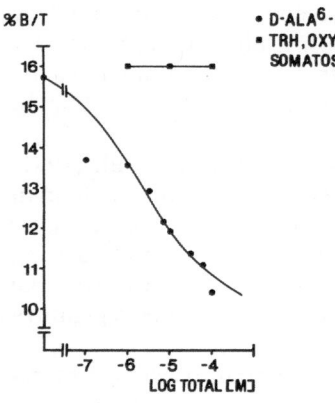

Fig. 2. Displacement of ^{125}I-labeled [D-Ala^6-desGly^{10}]-LH-RH ethylamide from membranes of a well-differentiated serous papillary adenocarcinoma by increasing concentrations of cold LH-RH analog and other peptides. Thyrotropin-releasing hormone (*TRH*), oxytocin, somatostatin and corticotropin-releasing factor (*CRF*) did not displace the binding. (From Emons et al. 1989, with permission from Pergamon Press)

carcinomata (Table 1). The analysis of the binding data obtained from inhibition curves with unlabeled LH-RH analogs was consistent with a single class of low-affinity, high-capacity binding sites ($K_a = 1.42 \times 10^5$ l/mol; $B_{max} = 209 \pm 69 \times 10^{-12}$ M/mg membrane protein; $n = 32$) (Emons et al. 1989). Oxytocin, thyrotropin-releasing hormone, and corticotropin-releasing hormone did not cause any displacement of ^{125}I-labeled LH-RH agonist. In contrast, somatostatin showed cross-reactivity in some of the tumors tested, whereas it did not displace the LH-RH agonist in others (Fig. 2). Native LH-RH, other LH-RH agonists, and some LH-RH antagonists were bound with nearly the same characteristics as [D-Ala^6-desGly^{10}]-LH-RH ethylamide. Of the 40 ovarian cancers tested, specific LH-RH-agonist binding could be demonstrated in 32 (Emons et al. 1989).

Using a photoaffinity labeling technique and subsequent sodium dodecyl sulfate-polyacrylamide gel electrophoresis, we could identify a specific high

Table 2. Molecular weights of LH-RH-binding sites labeled with ^{125}I [D-Lys^6-N^ε-azidobenzoyl]-LH-RH after Sodium dodecyl sulfate polyacrylamide gel electrophoresis and autoradiography. (From Pahwa et al. 1989, with permission from Academic Press)

Material	High-molecular weight component ($\times 10^3$ dalton)[a]	Low-molecular weight component ($\times 10^3$ dalton)[b]
Poorly to middle grade differentiated adenocarcinoma	64.5	45.5
Papillary adenocarcinoma	64.5	47.8
Partly solid, partly papillary carcinoma	64.5	n.d.
Poorly differentiated, predominantly solid cystadenocarcinoma	58.5	47.0[c]
Poorly differentiated, partly papillary adenocarcinoma	62.5	43.0[d]
Middle grade to highly differentiated adenocarcinoma	64.5	46.5

n.d., not detected.
[a] Mean ± SE 63.2 ± 0.99.
[b] Mean ± SE 46.0 ± 0.830.
[c] Mean value; range 45.5–48.5.
[d] Mean value; range 41.5–44.5.

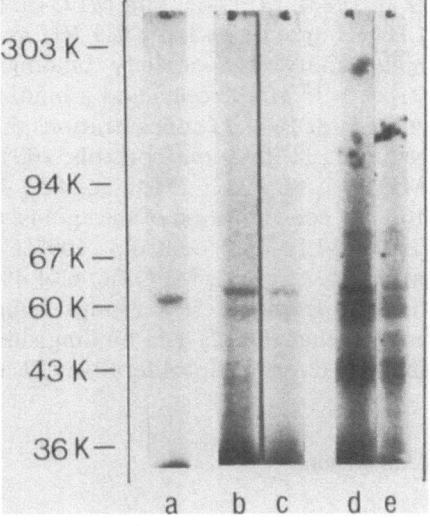

Fig. 3. Autoradiograms of sodium dodecyl sulfate-polyacrylamide gel electrophoresis of [^{125}I, D-Lys^6-N^ε-azidobenzoyl]-LH-RH labeled rat pituitary membranes (*a*). Plasma membranes prepared from a partly solid, partly papillary ovarian carcinoma in the absence (*b*) and presence (*c*) of 10^{-4} *M* [D-Ala^6-desGly^{10}]-LH-RH ethylamide. Plasma membranes prepared from a papillary adenocarcinoma in the absence (*d*) and presence (*e*) of 10^{-4} *M* LH-RH ethylamide. (From Pahwa et al. 1989, with permission from Academic Press)

molecular mass (63.3 kDa) binding site for LH-RH in human ovarian cancer. In addition, a smaller, less specific component of 46 kDa was present in some tumors, probably representing a degradation product of the specific binding site (Fig. 3, Table 2) (Pahwa et al. 1989). Skralovic, Schally and colleagues have recently also found a specific binding site for an LH-RH agonist in 29 out of 37 ovarian cancers. Using ^{125}I-labeled [D-Trp^6]-LH-RH, an analog with higher affinity than [D-Ala^6-desGly^{10}]-LH-RH ethylamide, they discriminated a high-affinity, low-capacity binding site and one of low affinity and high capacity (A. V. Schally, personal communication). The functional role of these LH-RH binding sites remains to be established. With three ovarian cancer cell lines (OVC NOVA, OV 166 and OV 1225) and the LH-RH agonist buserelin, Slotman et al. (1989) observed only minor but significant direct inhibitory effects on tumor cell proliferation.

Ohtani et al. (1990) recently reported that the in vitro proliferation of the ovarian adenocarcinoma cell lines HR, KF, and KFR was markedly stimulated by treatment with hCG and hMG. This increment in cell numbers was completely inhibited by treatment with the gonadotropin-releasing hormone (GnRH) agonist buserelin. All cell lines showed specific binding of ^{125}I-labeled FSH which decreased during buserelin treatment, indicating that the LH-RH agonist might act via a reduction of gonadotropin receptors. Thompson et al. (1991) found a dose-dependent retardation of the proliferation of the ovarian cancer cell line 2774 induced by the LH-RH agonist leuprolide. Flow cytometric cell cycle phase DNA analysis demonstrated that leuprolide caused a reversible 5%–6% increase in the portion of cells in G_0/G_1 phase, compared with controls during logarithmic growth, and a corresponding decrease in the portion of cells in DNA synthesis.

We recently studied four ovarian cancer cell lines, EFO-21, EFO-27 (Simon et al. 1983), MFO-35, and MFO-36 (Hofmann et al. 1989). Using the potent LH-RH agonist [D-Trp^6]-LH-RH as a radiolabel, we found in all cell lines a high-affinity, low-capacity binding site ($K_D = 8$–0.3×10^{-9} M; $B_{max} = 2$–31×10^{-15} $M/10^6$ cells) and a binding site of low affinity and high capacity. Already at 10^{-9} M concentrations the LH-RH agonist significantly ($p < 0.05$) reduced proliferation (controls, 100%; EFO-21, 88 ± 2%; EFO-27, 86 ± 4%; MFO-35, 86 ± 3%; MFO-36, 88 ± 4%). Growth inhibition increased with 10^{-7} M concentration of the agonist and was maximal ($p < 0.01$) at 10^{-5} M of [D-Trp^6]-LH-RH (controls, 100%; EFO-21, 66 ± 3%; EFO-27, 68 ± 3%; MFO-35, 65 ± 3%; MFO-36, 68 ± 4%) (Emons et al., in preparation). These findings from different groups using a variety of ovarian cancer cell lines suggest that the LH-RH binding sites found in human ovarian cancer might mediate direct antiproliferative effects of LH-RH agonists.

Conclusions

Considerable epidemiological and experimental data favor the hypothesis that ovarian cancer might be gonadotropin dependent. This hypothesis, however, cannot be accepted as an established fact yet, as there are contradictory findings that have to be taken into account. The important issue of whether or not ovarian cancers contain receptors for LH and/or FSH has to be settled.

The findings that gonadotropin preparations can contain contaminations with growth factors that stimulate the proliferation of ovarian cancer deserves great attention. The interpretation of mitogenic effects of gonadotropins on cancer cells must be conducted very carefully. Future experiments using go-nadotropin preparations purified from growth factor contaminations should clarify this issue.

The recent experiments on the growth promoting effects of castration on heterotransplanted human ovarian cancers in the nude mouse and the inhibi-tion of proliferation in the same model by suppressing gonadotropins with LH-RH agonists (Peterson and Zimniski 1990; Pour et al. 1988) strongly support the notion of a gonadotropin dependence of ovarian cancer. More experiments of this kind should be performed. The phase II clinical trials on LH-RH agonist induced gonadotropin suppression in ovarian cancer patients have also provided encouraging results. They have, however, to be evaluated by placebo-controlled trials.

The issue of direct LH-RH-analog effects on extrapituitary tissues has gained much attention during the last years. Not only for the human placenta and breast cancer (see introduction) but also for cancer of the prostate (Qayum et al. 1990 a, b), the pancreas (Fekete et al. 1989 b), and the endometrium (Srkalovic et al. 1990; Pahwa et al. 1991) data have been obtained which suggest autocrine regulatory systems based on LH-RH or a related compound.

As specified above, a substantial body of data has been obtained, indicating that such a system might also exist in ovarian cancer. We are, however, still far away from producing conclusive evidence for this hypothesis. The demonstra-tion of the production of LH-RH or a related compound in ovarian cancer cells is warranted. Also the LH-RH- or LH-RH-analog-induced activation of the classical LH-RH second messenger system (Naor 1990) in ovarian cancer cells has to be positively detected. A possible activation of tyrosine phos-phatases counteracting the effect of growth factors in the tumor cells should also be considered (Lee et al. 1991).

Additionally the question of the nature of the LH-RH binding sites (low-affinity, high-capacity and/or high-affinity/low-capacity) has to be answered by future research. Even if an autocrine system in ovarian cancer based on LH-RH or a related compound could be proven beyond any doubt, another problem had to be solved; namely, can we obtain sufficiently high concentra-tions of LH-RH analogs at the tumor cells in vivo to take advantage of possible direct inhibitory effects? This question would be especially relevant if the essential receptors should turn out to be the low-affinity/high-capacity type. In this case, new LH-RH analogs with high affinity to the extrapituitary binding sites ought to be developed before a therapeutic application is possi-ble.

An interesting alternative, which makes use even of the low-affinity binding sites for LH-RH in ovarian cancer, has been proposed by A. V. Schally's group. Analogs of LH-RH containing cytotoxic groups might be used for targeted chemotherapy (Bajusz et al. 1989 a, b). Future experiments will have to reveal if this approach is effective in vivo.

In conclusion, the facts available today are still far from providing convinc-ing evidence that ovarian cancer is gonadotropin dependent and/or that there are direct effects of LH-RH analogs on ovarian cancer. The data obtained so far, however, are already good enough to encourage intensive research in these fields which might open novel therapeutic approaches. Regarding the present unsatisfying situation in the treatment of advanced ovarian cancer and the relative standstill in the development of surgery, chemotherapy, and radiotherapy, an effective and nontoxic endocrine treatment for this malignancy would represent relevant progress.

Acknowledgements. Our work was supported by the Stiftung P. E. Kempkes, the Alfred and Ursula Kuhlemann-Stiftung (both Marburg) and Ferring Arzneimittel GmbH, Kiel, FRG. G. S. Pahwa was an Alexander von Humboldt fellow, on deputation from Regional Research Laboratory, Jammu Tawi, India.

References

Aten A, Polan ML, Bayless R, Behrman H (1987) A gonadotropin-releasing hormone (GnRH)-like protein in human ovaries: similarity to the GnRH-like ovarian protein of the rat. J Clin Endocrinol Metab 64:1288–1293

Averette HE, Donato DM (1990) Ovarian carcinoma, advances in diagnosis, staging and treatment. Cancer 65:703–708

Bajusz S, Janaky T, Csernus VJ, Bokser L, Fekete M, Srkalovic G, Redding TW, Schally AV (1989a) Highly potent metallopeptide analogues of luteinizing hormone-releasing hormone. Proc Natl Acad Sci USA 86:6313–6317

Bajusz S, Janaky T, Csernus VJ, Bokser L, Fekete M, Srkalovic G, Redding TW, Schally AV (1989b) Highly potent analogues of luteinizing hormone-releasing hormone containing D-phenylalanine nitrogen mustard in position 6. Proc Natl Acad Sci USA 86:6318–6322

Bauknecht T, Runge M, Schwall M, Pfleiderer A (1988) Occurrence of epidermal growth factor receptors (EGF-R) in human adnexal tumors and their prognostic value in advanced ovarian carcinomas. Gynecol Oncol 29:147–157

Belisle S, Guevin JF, Bellabarba D, Lehoux JG (1984) Luteinizing hormone releasing hormone binds to enriched placental membranes and stimulates in vitro the synthesis of bioactive human chorionic gonadotropin. J Clin Endocrinol Metab 59:119–126

Blackledge G, Lawton FG (1989) Second Birmingham gynecological cancer workshop on second line treatment of ovarian cancer. Br J Cancer 59:657–659

Blankenstein MA, Henkelman MS, Klijn JGM (1985) Direct inhibitory effect of a luteinizing hormone-releasing hormone agonist on MCF-7 human breast cancer cells. Eur J Cancer Clin Oncol 21:1493–1499

Bramley TA, Menzies GS, Baird DT (1985) Specific binding of gonadotropin-releasing hormone and an agonist to human corpus luteum homogenates: characterization, properties and luteal phase levels. J Clin Endocrinol Metab 61:834–841

Bruckner HW, Motwani BT (1989) Treatment of advanced refractory ovarian carcinoma with a gonadotropin-releasing hormone analogue. Am J Obstet Gynecol 161:1216–1218

Bützow R, Huhtaniemi I, Clayton R, Wahlström T, Andersson LC, Seppälä M (1987) Cultured mammary carcinoma cells contain gonadotropin releasing hormone-like immunoreactivity, GnRH binding sites and chorionic gonadotropin. Int J Cancer 39:498–501

Casagrande JT, Louie EW, Pike MC, Roy S, Rock RK, Henderson BE (1979) Incessant ovulation and ovarian cancer? Lancet 2:170–173

Casper RF, Erickson GF, Rebar RW, Yen SSC (1982) The effect of luteinizing hormone-releasing factor and its agonist on cultured human granulosa cells. Fertil Steril 37:406–409

Clayton RN, Huhtaniemi I (1982) Absence of gonadotropin-releasing hormone receptors in human gonadal tissue. Nature 299:56–59

Cramer DW, Welch WR (1983) Determinants of ovarian cancer risk: II. Inferences regarding pathogenesis. JNCI 71:717–721

Currie AJ, Fraser HM, Sharpe RM (1981) Human placental receptors for luteinizing hormone releasing hormone. Biochem Biophys Res Commun 89:332–338

Desombre ER, Holt JA, Herbst AC (1987) Steroid receptors in breast, uterine and ovarian malignancy. In: Gold JJ, Josinovich JB (eds) Gynecologic endocrinology. Plenum, New York, pp 511–528

Eidne KA, Flanagan CA, Harris NS, Millar RP (1987) Gonadotropin-releasing hormone (GnRH)-binding sites in human breast cancer cell lines and inhibitory effects of GnRH-antagonists. J Clin Endocrinol Metab 64:425–432

Emons G, Pahwa GS, Brack C, Sturm R, Oberheuser F, Knuppen R (1989) Gonadotropin-releasing hormone binding sites in human epithelial ovarian carcinomata. Eur J Cancer Clin Oncol 25:215–221

Emons G, Pahwa GS, Sturm R, Knuppen R, Oberheuser F (1990) The use of GnRH analogues in ovarian cancer. In: Vickery BH, Lunenfeld B (eds) GnRH analogues in cancer and human reproduction, vol 3. Kluwer, Dordrecht, pp 159–170

Fathalla MF (1971) Incessant ovulation – a factor in ovarian neoplasia? Lancet 2:163

Fekete M, Bajusz S, Groot K, Csernus VJ, Schally AV (1989a) Comparison of different agonists and antagonists of luteinizing hormone-releasing hormone for receptor-binding ability to rat pituitary and human breast cancer membranes. Endocrinology 124:946–955

Fekete M, Zalatnai A, Comaru-Schally AM, Schally AV (1989b) Membrane receptors for peptides in experimental and human pancreatic cancers. Pancreas 4:521–528

Freedman RS, Saul PS, Edwards CL, Jolles CJ, Gershenson DM, Jones LA, Atkinson EN, Dana WJ (1986) Ethinyl estradiol and medroxyprogesterone acetate in patients with epithelial ovarian carcinoma: a phase II study. Cancer Treat Rep 70:369–373

Hofmann J, Hölzel F, Hackenberg R, Schulz KD (1989) Characterization of epidermal growth-factor related proteins from human urinary chorionic gonadotropin. J Endocrinol 123:333–340

Hsueh AJW, Schaeffer M (1985) Gonadotropin-releasing hormone as a paracrine hormone and neurotransmitter in extrapituitary sites. J Steroid Biochem 23:757–764

Iwashita M, Evans MI, Catt KJ (1986) Characterization of a gonadotropin-releasing hormone receptor site in term placenta and chorionic villi. J Clin Endocrinol Metab 62:127–133

Jäger W, Wildt L, Lang N (1989) Some observations on the effects of a GnRH analog in ovarian cancer. Eur J Obstet Gynecol Reprod Biol 32:137–148

Kaldor JM, Day NE, Petterson F, Clarke EA, Pedersen D, Mehnert W, Bell J, Høst H, Prior P, Karjalainen S, Neal F, Koch M, Band P, Choi W, Kirn VP, Arslan A, Zarén B, Belch AR, Storm H, Kittelmann B, Fraser P, Stovall M (1990) Leukemia following chemotherapy for ovarian cancer. N Engl J Med 322:1–6

Kammerman S, Demopoulos RI, Raphael C, Ross J (1981) Gonadotropic hormone binding to human ovarian tumors. Hum Pathol 12:886–890

Kauppila A, Martikainen H, Pentinen J, Reinilä M (1990) GnRH-agonist analogue treatment of ovarian granulosa cell malignancies. Gynecol Endocrinol 4 [Suppl 2]:97

Kavanagh JJ, Roberts W, Townsend P, Hewitt S (1989) Leuprolide acetate in the treatment of refractory or persistent epithelial ovarian cancer. J Clin Oncol 7:115–118

Knecht M, Ranta T, Feng P, Shinohara O, Catt KJ (1985) Gonadotropin-releasing hormone as a modulator of ovarian function. J Steroid Biochem 23:771–778

Kullander S, Rausing A, Schally AV (1987) LH-RH agonist treatment in ovarian cancer. In: Klijn JGM (ed) Hormonal manipulation of cancer: peptides, growth factors and new (anti) steroidal agents. Raven, New York, pp 353–356

Kvale G, Heuch J, Nilssen S, Beral V (1988) Reproductive factors and risk of ovarian cancer: a prospective study. Int J Cancer 42:246–251

Lamberts SWJ, Timmers JM, Oosterom R, Verleun T, Rommerts FG, de Jong FH (1982) Testosterone secretion by cultured arrhenoblastoma cells: suppression by a luteinizing hormone-releasing hormone agonist. J Clin Endocrinol Metab 54:450–454

Latouche J, Crumeyrolle-Arias M, Jordan D, Kopp N, Augendre-Ferrante B, Cedard L, Haour F (1991) GnRH receptors in human granulosa cells: anatomical localization and characterization by autoradiographic study. Endocrinology 125:1739–1741

Lee MT, Liebow C, Kramer AR, Schally AV (1991) Effects of epidermal growth factor and analogues of luteinizing hormone-releasing hormone and somatostatin on phosphorylation and dephosphorylation of tyrosine residues of specific protein substrates in various tumors. Proc Natl Acad Sci USA 88:1656–1660

Levy J, Segal T, Wiznitzer A, Insler V, Sharoni Y (1989) Molecular mechanisms of GnRH action on mammary tumors and uterine leiomyomata. In: Vickery BH, Lunenfeld B (eds) GnRH-Analogues in cancer and human reproduction, vol 1. Kluwer, Dordrecht, pp 127–136

Li CH, Ramasharma K, Yamashiro D, Chung D (1987) Gonadotropin-releasing peptide from human follicular fluid: isolation, characterization and chemical synthesis. Proc Natl Acad Sci USA 86:959–962

Mayer A (1925) Klinik der Ovarialtumoren, Ätiologie. In: Halban J, Seitz L (eds) Biologie und Pathologie des Weibes, vol 5, part 2. Urban und Schwarzenberg, München, pp 877–881

Miller WR, Scott WN, Morris R, Fraser HM, Sharpe RM (1985) Growth of human breast cancer cells inhibited by a luteinizing hormone-releasing hormone agonist. Nature 313:231–233

Mortel R, Satyaswaroop PG, Schally AV, Hamilton T, Ozols R (1986) Inhibitory effect of GnRH superagonist on the growth of human ovarian carcinoma NIH: OVCAR 3 in the nude mouse. Gynecol Oncol 23:254–255

MRC Gynecologic Cancer Working Party (1990) An overview in the treatment of advanced ovarian cancer. Br J Cancer 61:495–496

Mullen P, Scott WN, Miller WR (1991) Growth inhibition observed following administration of an LH-RH agonist to a clonal variant of the MCF-7 breast cancer cell line is accompanied by an accumulation of cells in the G0/G1 phase of the cell cycle. Br J Cancer 63:930–932

Nakano R, Kitayama S, Yamoto M, Ooshima A (1989) Localization of gonadotropin binding sites in human ovarian neoplasms. Am J Obstet Gynecol 161:905–910

Naor Z (1990) Signal transduction mechanisms of Ca^{2+} mobilizing hormones: the case of gonadotropin-releasing hormone. Endocr Rev 11:326–353

Ohtani K (1990) Effects of gonadotropin on the growth of malignant ovarian neoplasms assessed by subrenal capsule assay. Nippon Sanka Fujinka Gakki Zasshi 42:579–585

Ohtani K, Sakamoto H, Konbai D (1990) Antagonistic effects of GnRH agonist on gonadotropin stimulated proliferation of human ovarian cancer cell line. Gynecol Endocrinol 4 (Suppl 2):98

Olshausen R (1877) Die Krankheiten der Ovarien, Ätiologie. In: Billroth T (ed) Handbuch der Frauenkrankheiten, vol 6. Enke, Stuttgart, pp 74–78

Olsson JH, Akesson I, Hillensjoe T (1990) Effects of a gonadotropin-releasing hormone agonist on progesterone formation in cultured human granulosa cells. Acta Endocrinol (Copenh) 122:427–431

Pahwa GS, Vollmer G, Knuppen R, Emons G (1989) Photoaffinity labelling of gonadotropin releasing hormone binding sites in human epithelial ovarian carcinomata. Biochem Biophys Res Commun 161:1086–1092

Pahwa GS, Kullander S, Vollmer G, Oberheuser F, Knuppen R, Emons G (1991) Specific low affinity binding sites for gonadotropin releasing hormone in human endometrial carcinomata. Eur J Obstet Gynecol Reprod Biol 41:135–142

Parmar H, Nicoll J, Stockdale A, Cassoni A, Phillips RH, Lightman SL, Schally AV (1985) Advanced ovarian carcinoma: response to the agonist D-Trp[6]-LH-RH. Cancer Treat Rep 69:1341–1342

Parmar H, Phillips RH, Rustin F, Lightman SL, Hanham JW, Schally AV (1988a) Therapy of advanced ovarian cancer with D-Trp[6]-LH-RH (decapeptyl) microcapsules. Biomed Pharmacother 42:531–538

Parmar H, Rustin F, Lightman SL, Phillips RH, Hanham JW, Schally AV (1988 b) Response to D-Trp[6]-luteinizing hormone releasing hormone (Decapeptyl) microcapsules in advanced ovarian cancer. B M J 296:1229

Pellicer A, Miró F (1990) Steroidogenesis in vitro of human granulosa-luteal cells pretreated in vivo with gonadotropin-releasing hormone analogs. Fertil Steril 54:590–596

Peterson CM, Zimniski SJ (1990) A long acting gonadotropin-releasing hormone agonist inhibits the growth of a human ovarian epithelial carcinoma (BG-1) heterotransplanted in the nude mouse. Obstet Gynecol 76:264–267

Petraglia F, Vaughan J, Vale W (1990) Steroid hormones modulate the release of immunoreactive gonadotropin-releasing hormone from cultured human placental cells. J Clin Endocrinol Metab 70:1173–1178

Popkin R, Bramley TA, Currie A, Shaw RW, Baird DT, Fraser HM (1983) Specific binding of luteinizing hormone-releasing hormone to human luteal tissue. Biochem Biophys Res Commun 114:750–756

Pour PM, Redding TW, Paz-Bouza JI, Schally AV (1988) Treatment of experimental ovarian carcinoma with monthly injection of the agonist D-Trp[6]-LH-RH: a preliminary report. Cancer Lett 41:105–110

Qayum A, Gullick W, Clayton RC, Sikora K, Waxman J (1990a) The effects of gonadotropin-releasing hormone analogues in prostate cancer are mediated through specific tumour receptors. Br J Cancer 62:96–99

Qayum A, Gullick WJ, Mellon K, Krausz T, Neal D, Sikora K, Waxman J (1990b) The partial purification and characterization of the GnRH-like activity from prostatic biopsy specimens and prostatic cancer cell lines. J Steroid Biochem Mol Biol 37:899–902

Radovick S, Wondisford FE, Nakayama Y, Yamada M, Cutler GB Jr, Weintraub BD (1990) Isolation and characterization of the human gonadotropin-releasing hormone gene in the hypothalamus and placenta. Mol Endocrinol 4:476–480

Rajaniemi H, Kauppila A, Rönnberg L, Selander K, Pystynen P (1981) LH (hCG) receptor in benign and malignant tumors of human ovary. Acta Obstet Gynecol Scand Suppl 101:83–86

Rao BR, Slotman BJ (1991) Endocrine factors in common epithelial ovarian cancer. Endocr Rev 12:14–26

Scambia G, Panici PB, Baiocchi G, Perrone L, Gaggini G, Iacobelli S, Mancuso S (1988) Growth inhibitory effect of LH-RH analogs on human breast cancer cells. Anticancer Res 8:187–190

Schlesselman JJ (1989) Cancer of the breast and reproductive tract in relation to use of oral contraceptives. Contraception 40:1–38

Seppälä M, Wahlström R (1980) Identification of luteinizing hormone releasing factor and α-subunit of glycoprotein hormones in ductal carcinoma of the mammary gland. Int J Cancer 26:231–233

Siler-Khodr TM, Khodr GS (1980) Placental luteinizing hormone releasing factor and its synthesis. Science 207:315–317

Simon WE, Hölzel F (1979) Hormone sensitivity of gynecological tumor cells in tissue cultures. J Cancer Res Clin Oncol 94:307–323

Simon WE, Albrecht M, Hänsel M, Dietl M, Hölzel F (1983) Cell lines derived from human ovarian carcinomas: growth stimulation by gonadotropic and steroid hormones. JNCI 70:839–845

Slotman BJ, Poels LG, Rao BR (1989) A direct LH-RH-agonist action on cancer cells is unlikely to be the cause of response to LH-RH-agonist treatment. Anticancer Res 9:77–80

Srkalovic G, Wittliff JL, Schally AV (1990) Detection and partial characterization of receptors for [D-Trp[6]]-luteinizing hormone-releasing hormone and epidermal growth factor in human endometrial carcinoma. Cancer Res 50:1841–1846. Erratum published in: Cancer Res 50:3808

Stadel BV (1975) The etiology and prevention of ovarian cancer. Am J Obstet Gynecol 123:772–774

Stouffer RL, Grodin MS, Davis JR, Surwitt EA (1984) Investigation of binding sites for follicle-stimulating hormone and chorionic gonadotropin in human ovarian cancers. J Clin Endocrinol Metab 59:441–446

Tan GJS, Biggs JSG (1983) Absence of effect of LH-RH on progesterone production by human luteal cells in vitro. J Reprod Fertil 67:411–413

Thompson MA, Adelson MD, Kaufman LM (1991) Lupron retards proliferation of ovarian epithelial tumor cells cultured in serum-free medium. J Clin Endocrinol Metab 72:1036–1041

Tureck RW, Mastroianni L Jr, Blasco L, Strauß JF III (1982) Inhibition of human granulosa cell progesterone secretion by a gonadotropin-releasing hormone agonist. J Clin Endocrinol Metab 54:1078–1080

Wilding C, Chen M, Gelman EP (1987) LH-RH agonists and human breast cancer cells. Nature 329:770

Treatment of Endometrial Cancer with GnRH Analogs

S. Kullander

Department of Obstetrics and Gynecology, General Hospital, 21401 Malmö, Sweden

Introduction

In many Western countries, endometrial carcinoma is now considered to be the most common gynecological malignancy, but mortality from this disease is less than that for ovarian malignancies. Nearly 20% of patients with endometrial carcinoma get second primaries, mostly in the breast and colon, indicating common denominators for many of these tumors. Certain factors predispose to this cancer. Many patients are obese, nulliparous, and have a history of irregular menses suggesting a basic abnormality in the hypothalamic-pituitary-ovarian hormonal axis. Long periods of unopposed estrogen stimulation of the endometrium may be a factor in carcinogenesis, since the endometrium is a highly sensitive end-organ to estrogens, regardless of whether they are of gonadal origin or exogenously administered. When the estrogen-induced growth is unopposed by progesterone (due to a lack of ovulations or for other reasons) the endometrium first shows hyperplasia. If the epithelial activity is excessive, adenomatous hyperplasia with prominent mitoses and changes that are difficult to distinguish from frank adenocarcinoma appear. The risk factors are also shared by these two conditions. Although treatment with progesterones may in some cases reverse an adenomatous hyperplasia so that even a desired pregnancy will be possible, in the somewhat older woman hysterectomy is considered to be the safest approach. In particular, the presence of cytonuclear atypia raises concern for premalignancy and progression to cancer. It has also been proposed that such lesions should be referred to as endometrial intraepithelial neoplasia (EIN).

The real, invasive carcinoma is distinguished by the stromal invasion. Most patients with endometrial cancer have no evidence of spread beyond the body of the uterus. The uterus may often be larger than average for the patient's age and parity. As myomas are common in such patients, a co-incidence with endometrial carcinoma is not uncommon and also often contributes to an enlarged uterus. Menorrhagia in this cancer may lead to secondary anemia. Besides the general physical state of the patient (affected by, for example, age, diabetes, or hypertension), which may contraindicate surgery, several other factors influence treatment decisions. An enlarged uterus probably indicates a poorer prognosis and increases operative risks. An increasing depth of penetration through the myometrium and a poorly differentiated adenocarcinoma are also unfavorable. Undifferentiated adenocarcinomas often lack sex-steroid receptors.

In management of the disease, conservative hysterectomy is the corner-stone of treatment in an otherwise healthy woman. Where there is regional spread, additional radiation is used. Hormonal gestagen therapy is considered of value especially for patients with generalized disease. At present, cytotoxic chemotherapy has no defined place in the primary management of the disease. Gestagens have been used extensively, and responders, probably those with receptors for the hormone, sometimes achieve long-term survival. Side effects, however, do occur, especially at high doses, and include fluid retentions and allergic reactions as well as cardiovascular events. It follows logically from the considerable body of evidence that genesis and growth of endometrial cancer may be estrogen-dependent and the proven presence of estrogen receptors in many of these tumors that suppression of intrinsic estrogen production by gonadotropin-releasing hormone (GnRH) agonists might be therapeutically valuable. Some clinical observations have as a matter of fact also shown that the use of GnRH agonists can lead to remission or stable disease in patients with advanced endometrial cancer. The first report on the effects of luteinizing hormone releasing hormone (LH-RH) agonists administered to a patient with endometrial carcinoma appeared in 1987 (Perl et al. 1987). A 36-year-old woman with obesity and a long history of infertility due to anovulatory cycles developed an atypical adenomatous hyperplasia of the endometrium with transition to adenocarcinoma. Eighty days of treatment with medroxyprogesterone acetate (MPA) did not alter the histological picture. However, following 3 months of therapy with an agonist, mitoses were no longer seen, but there were signs of differentiation in the tumor biopsy. In 1990, Gallagher et al. reported on 11 postmenopausal patients with recurrent endometrial cancer after surgery, radiotherapy, and treatment with MPA, who were treated with an LH-RH analog. In all of them, gonadotropins were suppressed and remission was achieved in five patients for up to 24 months; three patients had stable disease for up to 12 months.

More controlled clinical studies are necessary, however, to assess the efficacy of GnRH agonist treatment alone or in addition to conventional surgery and radiotherapy. A protocol for a multicenter clinical trial both for first-line treatment and for second-line should cover the points outlined in the following.

Clinical Aspects

The aim of a phase II clinical trial investigating GnRH agonists in endometrial cancer should be to answer the questions whether GnRH agonists are effective in the treatment of endometrial cancer, and what side effects are.

First-line therapy should be conducted in the specific interval between primary diagnosis by curettage and primary surgical treatment. The *admission criterion* should be endometrial carcinoma, diagnosed by sharp curettage (histology). The projected number of patients is 10–20.

A second line of therapy should be GnRH agonist treatment in advanced cases of endometrial cancer. Here patients should be included who have advanced or relapsed endometrial cancer which is refractory to conventional surgery, irradiation, and cytotoxic chemotherapy or in patients who refuse or do not tolerate chemotherapy. Endometrial cancer must be diagnosed histologically. No other endocrine or cytotoxic or irradiation therapy should be used during the trial. The projected number of patients is 30.

Parameters which should be assessed at the beginning of treatment are age, weight, menopausal age, hemoglobin, and erythrocyte sedimentation rate. Ten milliliters of deep-frozen serum in 2-ml portions should be stored for later hormone and tumor marker analyses. Size of tumor and/or metastases should be determined by palpation and, if possible, by image generating techniques such as computed tomography or sonography. Conventional chest X-ray should be performed. The same parameters and remission status should then be assessed at 2-month intervals and tumor biopsies, if available, should be examined histologically. Patients should be treated with monthly injections of an agonist depot preparation until progression, death, or severe side effects occur.

Case Report

Adenomatous hyperplasia could be used instead of endometrial carcinoma for first-line therapy as suggested by Perl et al. (1987). I have personally observed a case similar to Perl et al.'s (1987). A 26-year-old nulliparous woman had irregular and heavy menstruations since menarche at 16 years, and in the previous 2 years she also had inter-menstrual bleedings. She did not tolerate gestagen. Serum estradiol (E_2) was 0.75 nmol/l, and luteinizing hormone (LH) 2.6 IU/l. At curettage, adenomatous hyperplasia with grave atypia, possibly highly differentiated adenocarcinoma was found and it was proposed that hysterectomy should be considered. Agonist treatment was started and 4 weeks later E_2 was 0.05 nmol/l; 3 months later follicle-stimulating hormone (FSH) was 1.4 IU/l and $E_2 < 0.04$ nmol/l. Sonography after 4 months of treatment showed a thin atrophic endometrium. Curettage now showed fragments of an inactive endometrium with highly differentiated cylindric epithelium. Treatment therefore was stopped. Normal menstruations reappeared and now the patient would like to have a child.

Discussion

In addition to alterations in hormone profiles, it also seems possible that GnRH analogs have direct effects on endometrial cancer. Specific GnRH-binding sites have been discovered and partially characterized in endometrial cancer by two groups (Emons et al. 1988; Srkalovic et al. 1990). Emons et al. (1988) and Pahwa et al. (1990) found them very similar to other human extra-pituitary GnRH-binding sites of the low affinity and high capacity type, e.g., in breast cancer and ovarian cancer. GnRH binding could be demonstrated in all 12 endometrial tumor samples tested. A photolabeled derivative of GnRH was prepared, and photoaffinity labeling of endometrial carcinoma cell membranes and subsequent electrophoresis in polyacrylamide gel revealed a single molecular weight component of 62 kDa. The appearance of this photolabeled binding site could be suppressed by the addition of unlabeled GnRH agonist, but not by other peptides and is thus a specific binding site. Similar binding sites were also present in pooled endometrium from postmenopausal women. Those binding sites may be of physiological relevance as receptors for GnRH which are formed locally as part of an autocrine mechanism regulating normal endometrial growth.

The Schally group found specific binding in 24 out of 31 endometrial cancers and in 3 of 13 nonmalignant human endometrial biopsies. They also considered this finding a rationale for LH-RH analog therapy in this cancer.

It is not clear why some discrepancy in results was found by the Schally group (Srkalovic et al. 1990), which reported on a single class of high-affinity receptors in human endometrial carcinoma. A detailed analysis of the relation between binding affinity and histology (e.g., amounts of tumor cells in relation to stroma cells) is difficult on limited amounts of material, but could be essential for an explanating of the discrepancy. The use of different ligands and methods of separation could be one reason for it, but further experiments are needed to elucidate the matter.

The mucosal lining of endometriotic cysts may have GnRH-binding sites like those shown in normal endometrium. A similar local mechanism may then be operative in a successful treatment of endometriosis and endometrial cancer.

There are many studies indicating a reduction in uterine volume after treatment with GnRH agonists. The mechanism for this reduction in size is not known, but the induced suppression of estrogens may be one of the primary causes. Such an effect is of course favorable for the surgical treatment of a myomatous or an enlarged cancerous uterus. Changes in the local blood flow may be one cause of the regression processes. There are estrogen receptors in the pelvic vessel walls, and steroids are important for vessel diameter and vessel wall impedance. The new vaginal color Doppler technique is an excellent tool for studying blood flow dynamics in myomas, and ovarian and endometrial cancers. A low wall resistance index with increased blood flow, as is often seen in these tumors, must be favorable for the tumor growth. It would be of interest to follow the resistance index longitudinally under agonist treatment.

Summary

Given the small number of side effects, GnRH may be a useful and ideal drug for new therapeutic hormonal approaches in many cases of both invasive and noninvasive endometrial cancer. The hypoestrogenic state thus induced as well as a local effect may lead to pronounced regression of the tumor. Any future therapy should, however, always be tailored to meet individual needs. The use of GnRH agonists may be advocated in the following circumstances:

1. In pronounced endometrial hyperplasia and adenomatous hyperplasia (particularly relevant in those cases where hysterectomy is not desirable, e.g., in young patients who have not yet completed their families).
2. In patients with endometrial cancer where surgery is contraindicated or refused.
3. In addition to or as a substitute for radium treatment preoperatively to reduce uterine volume (myomas) to make surgery technically easier; to devitalize the tumor, stop menorrhagia, and improve anemia.
4. In advanced cases as an adjunct to radiotherapy and gestagens. It is possible that this will produce synergistic effects.
5. As adjuvant treatment (replacing gestagens?) in primary stages.
6. In relapses of endometrial cancer, refractory to conventional therapy, and in pulmonary metastases.

References

Emons G, Kullander S, Pahwa GS (1988) GnRH-binding in human endometrial cancer. Abstracts of the 12th world congress of gynecology and obstetrics, 23–28 October 1988, Rio de Janeiro, Brazil, p 560

Gallagher CJ, Oliver RTD, Hope-Stone HF, Oram D, Fowler C (1990) Proceeding of the 2nd international symposium on GnRH analogues in cancer and human reproduction, November 8–11, 1990, Geneva

Pahwa GS, Kullander S, Vollmer G, Oberheuser F, Knuppen R, Emons G (1991) Specific low affinity binding sites for gonadotropin releasing hormone in human endometrial carcinomata. Eur J Obstet Gynecol Reprod Biol 41:135–142

Perl V, Schally AV, Comaru-Schally AM, Marquez J, Dabancens A, Navarro C (1987) Use of D-Trp[6]-LH-RH in endometrial adenocarcinoma. 22nd congreso chileno de obstetricia y ginecologia, 1987, Santiago, vol 2

Srkalovic G, Wittliff JL, Schally AV (1990) Detection and partial characterization of receptors for D-Trp[6]-luteinizing hormone-releasing hormone and epidermal growth factor in human endometrial carcinoma. Cancer Res 50:1841–1846

LH-RH Agonists in the Treatment of Metastatic Breast Cancer: Ten Years' Experience

J. G. M. Klijn

Division of Endocrine Oncology, Department of Medical Oncology,
Rotterdam Cancer Institute (Dr. Daniel den Hoed Cancer Center), P.O. Box 5201,
3008 AE Rotterdam, The Netherlands

Introduction

Different steroid and peptide hormones, growth factors and other tropic substances are involved in the growth regulation of breast cancer cells. Estrogens play an especially important role. Since the observation of tumor growth remission after surgical castration by Beatson in 1896, various treatment modalities have been developed which suppress gonadal and/or peripheral estrogen production or which antagonize the stimulatory effects of estrogens at the level of the tumor cells [1, 2]. Apart from castration by surgical or radiotherapeutic means, it is possible to suppress pituitary-gonadal function by different kinds of medical treatment. In the past decade it became clinically apparent that luteinizing hormone releasing hormone (LH-RH) analogs are of great interest for suppressing pituitary-gonadal function in the treatment of metastatic breast and prostate cancer, especially because of the absence of serious side effects [3–6].

Since the unravelment of the structure of LH-RH and elucidation of its physiology by Schally and Guilemin (1971), numerous analogs with pronounced and long-term effects have been synthesized and tested [4–11]. Most of these agents appeared to have a paradoxical antifertility effect during long-term treatment with sufficiently high (supraphysiological) doses. The most potent of these analogs have been used in experimental and clinical studies.

In 1976, DeSombre et al. [12] reported for the first time regression of rat mammary tumors effected by an LH-RH analog. Since then a number of experimental studies on endocrine and growth inhibitory effects in rodents with different kinds of tumors have been published [4, 7–10, 13].

Summarizing these data, chronic LH-RH agonist treatment with pharmacological doses appears to cause:

1. "Partial hypophysectomy" with decreased gonadotropin and prolactin secretion

2. "Chemical castration" with a striking fall in plasma sex steroids followed by a reduction in weight of accessory sex organs
3. Inhibition of enzymes involved in steroidogenesis
4. Direct effects on extrapituitary tissues such as gonadal tissue and both breast and prostate tumor cells

In addition, the finding of the presence of LH-RH-like material and LH-RH receptors in experimental and human breast tumors, and of direct growth inhibitory effects on tumor cells in vitro (for reviews see [14] and Foekens and Klijn, this volume), stimulated performance of clinical trials. Ten years ago, in 1981, we started the first trial and reported preliminary results 1 year later [3]. Since then, a series of phase II studies have been carried out by several investigators using different LH-RH analogs and formulations [1, 5, 15]. The first large comparative phase III studies with LH-RH agonists are now at an advanced stage. Furthermore, new potent LH-RH antagonists are available for experimental studies and phase I trials [11, 16, 17]. In this report, we will shortly summarize the results of 10 years of clinical research with LH-RH analogs in breast cancer, focusing on our results with buserelin.

Dose and Mode of Administration

Initially, formulation was a problem. LH-RH and its analogs are small peptides susceptible to alimentary tract digestion and, therefore, unsuitable for oral use. Therefore, early clinical trials by us [3, 15, 18–24] and others [1, 5, 25–30] used nasal spray – buserelin – or daily subcutaneous – buserelin, leuprolide, Zoladex (goserelin) – or intramuscular – Decapeptyl (triptorelin) – injections. Later on, depot formulations of these analogs became available for clinical administration offering patients greater efficacy and much more comfort [1, 10, 11, 31–40].

During these studies, a great interindividual variation in endocrine response appeared. While there is relatively little difference in potency between the commonly used LH-RH analogs, some patients need 100 times higher dosages than others to reach complete "medical castration". In general, amenorrhea has been observed in 15%–20% of patients receiving a daily dose of 400–600 µg buserelin intranasally (equivalent to approximately 8–12 µg subcutaneously), in 40% treated with 1200 µg intranasally (approximately 25 µg subcutaneously), in approximately 75% treated with 100–1000 µg by daily subcutaneous injections and in 100% of the patients treated with approximately 1 mg in daily injections or with monthly depot preparations (approximately 3.6 mg per depot formulation). Relatively lower daily dosages between 50 and 300 µg can achieve medical castration in (nearly) all patients when administered continuously by infusion or slow-release formulations. On the other hand, the highest dosages may have the advantage of potential direct antitumor effects in vivo. In clinical practice, at present mainly depot preparations are being used in the treatment of breast cancer.

Pharmacokinetics in Relation to Endocrine Effects

The binding affinity of LH-RH agonists to pituitary LH-RH receptors is about ten times higher than that of the natural hormone LH-RH [41]. They are relatively resistant to degradation by pituitary enzymes, block the LH-RH receptors of the gonadotropic cells making them unresponsive to subsequent stimulation, and prevent pulsatile stimulation of the pituitary by hypothalamic LH-RH resulting in medical castration during long-term treatment [42, 43]. After administration of LH-RH agonists, there is a direct elimination of intact peptide into the urine and excretion of metabolites after hepatic inactivation. Buserelin is eliminated from plasma four times slower than natural LH-RH [42, 43]. Intranasal buserelin treatment caused lower plasma levels and lower urinary excretion of buserelin (7–20 μg/24 h) than two 1 mg injections daily (439 μg/24 h [42]). After subcutaneous injection or depot implantation, peak plasma concentrations of buserelin are reached after 30–60 min and 4–6 h, respectively. After intravenous injection, a rapid distribution phase is followed by a slower elimination phase with a plasma half-life of approximately 75–85 min. Protein binding of buserelin is about 15% [44]. Enzymes in liver and kidney degrade buserelin, and peptide metabolites are excreted and eliminated with bile or urine [41–44]. In the human, more than 30% of the dose administered is excreted in the urine. This peptide material consists of 55% intact buserelin and 32% of the (5–9) pentapeptide as the main metabolite.

In two clinical studies of six patients with mastalgia and ten patients with metastatic breast cancer (the latter group being also treated with tamoxifen) we investigated the relation between pharmacokinetics and endocrine effects of buserelin implants. In the patients with mastalgia, using single treatment with buserelin implants (polylactic glycol matrix, PLG, 50 : 50, 6.6 mg), there was an initial rise in plasma and urinary buserelin levels on the first treatment day followed by a rapid fall during the next 2 days [31–33]. After a plateau phase (60–80 μg/g creatinine), urinary buserelin/creatinine ratios decreased slowly to a mean value of 25 μg/g creatinine 4 weeks after implantation (Fig. 1).

Plasma estradiol concentrations dropped to castration values within 2 weeks of treatment, reaching a mean concentration of 17 pmol/l compared to 27 pmol/l ($p < 0.01$) determined in 680 postmenopausal control women [33]. After the last implant injection, urinary buserelin/creatinine ratios remained relatively high (over 5 ug/g creatinine) for more than 8 weeks followed by an exponential decrease (half-life of buserelin release = 15 days) to undetectable buserelin levels at 16–22 weeks after the last implantation. A rise of suppressed plasma estradiol concentrations to above castration levels was found 15–20 weeks after the last buserelin implantation, at a time when urinary buserelin excretion had decreased to below 0.2 μg/g creatinine [33]. It is concluded that after initial suppression of pituitary-ovarian function only very low concentrations of buserelin are needed to maintain suppression of ovarian activity by using slow-release preparations.

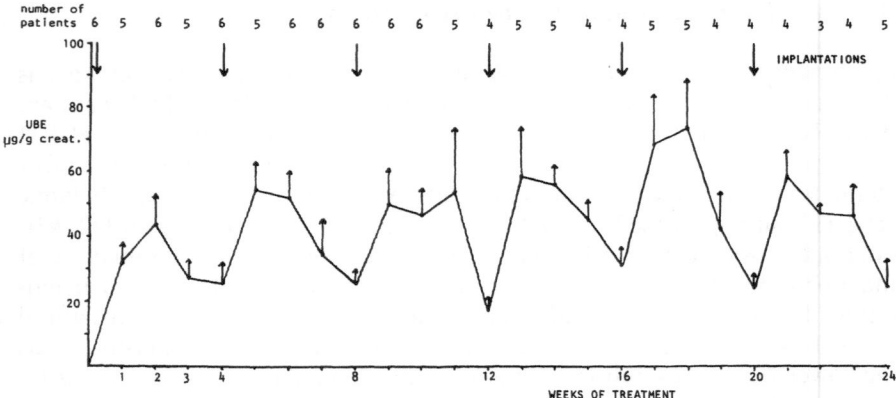

Fig. 1. Urinary buserelin excretion (*UBE*, mean ± SEM) during treatment with PLG 50 : 50 implants in six patients with mastalgia

The stimulatory effect of tamoxifen on pituitary-ovarian function [18, 45] counteract the suppressive effect of LH-RH agonist treatment [18–20]. Therefore, we studied endocrine and pharmacokinetic effects in a group of ten patients with metastatic breast cancer treated with buserelin implants in combination with tamoxifen (2 × 20 mg), to determine the level of buserelin which can prevent stimulation of the ovaries by tamoxifen. Pharmacokinetic studies showed that plasma concentrations of buserelin of (more than) 0.20 µg/ml resulting in urinary excretion of (more than) 5 µg/g creatinine after implantation of buserelin implants (once every 8 weeks) caused continuous suppression of pituitary-ovarian function in spite of the presence of tamoxifen [46].

Endocrine Effects

Premenopausal Patients

Previously, we reported extensively the endocrine effects observed in our studies with buserelin [3, 5, 18–24, 31–33]. In summary, on the first treatment day plasma gonadotropins reached peak values 4–6 h after start of single treatment with the LH-RH agonist [15, 21]. Thereafter follicle stimulating hormone (FSH) dropped more rapidly than LH to below pretreatment levels within 3 days and 2–3 weeks, respectively [19]. Anovulation, as indicated by persistent low plasma progesterone levels, occurred in all patients accompanied by a fall in plasma estradiol concentrations to castration levels within 2–4 weeks of treatment. Strikingly, during treatment with buserelin implants, plasma estradiol levels were significantly lower (17 pmol/l) at least during the first 3 months as compared with plasma estradiol concentrations observed in postmenopausal control (mean 27–34 pmol/l) [31, 33]. This is in agreement with the finding of Dowsett and Harris et al. who showed suppression of postmenopausal ovarian androgen secretion with Zoladex treatment, resulting in lower estrogen levels, i.e., a decrease from 33 to 22 pmol/l [47, 48].

With prolactin, on the first treatment day a small rise in plasma prolactin occurs, but this disappears during continuing treatment [15, 21]. Other authors have found no significant effect on basal prolactin levels [5] or a slight decrease [34]. We observed a significant decrease of the mean natural night peak of prolactin from 27.2 to 15.9 µg/l during chronic treatment [21].

In general, similar endocrine findings have been reported by other investigators. A disparity in the long-term effects on LH and FSH has been reported [1, 35, 38, 39] showing a rise of FSH and not of LH during chronic treatment. The reduction of circulating concentrations of estradiol is not influenced by patient age or weight [34, 35]. Plasma levels of estrone, androstenedione, and testosterone have been reported also to decrease (10%–30%) with LH-RH agonist therapy [35, 39], but cortisol levels are not affected [1]. Comparison of ovarian histology in primary oophorectomized and Zoladex-treated premenopausal patients has not revealed any gross abnormalities in the ovaries of long-term LH-RH agonist treated patients, but there was a significant reduction in the number of corpora lutea and a slight increase in the number of follicular cysts [49].

With respect to tumor estrogen receptor (ER) and progesterone receptor (PgR) levels, in rats with dimethylbenzanthracene (DMBA)-induced mammary tumors, we found a clear decrease in tumor steroid receptor content with buserelin therapy [22, 50], as was also observed after surgical castration [22].

Postmenopausal Patients

In postmenopausal patients plasma LH and FSH levels are also clearly suppressed by LH-RH agonist therapy [47, 48, 51, 53]. Some authors found no significant endocrine effect on plasma steroid levels [34, 51, 52], but Dowsett et al. [47] and Crighton et al. [53] demonstrated a significant fall in plasma androgen (substrate for peripheral conversion to estrogens) and estradiol levels (15%–22%). This discrepancy might be explained by technical differences between hormone assays, especially with respect to sensitivity for the lower limit of detection of estradiol. No significant effects on plasma prolactin level have been observed in postmenopausal women, but prolactin levels can markedly rise at the time of tumor progression as observed during other hormonal and cytotoxic treatments [53].

Antitumor Effects

Premenopausal Patients

Since the first study in 1981, we have treated more than 80 premenopausal patients with metastatic breast cancer within different trials, the last series within an ongoing EORTC phase III study (Fig. 2). The results in the first 46 patients are presented in Table 1. Twenty-three patients were treated with buserelin as single treatment, and 23 patients with combination therapy. The overall response rate is 39% with a median survival of 3 years, which is at least as good as has been reported for other kinds of endocrine therapy. The patients with combination treatment showed a somewhat better survival curve than the other patients, but the number is too small to draw definite conclusions [24]. Responding patients in our study and in other studies [26, 36–38] clearly showed longer survival than the nonresponders. One of our patients with the longest duration of response reported thus far, i.e., 5 years, has now survived for 10 years.

Similar results have been published by other investigators using different agonists (Table 2) [26–30, 37–39, 55–59]. In a total of 419 patients treated in 13 phase II studies, the response rate is exactly the same as that observed in our first study, i.e., 39%. There is no difference in efficacy between the various LH-RH agonists. Patients with ER-positive tumors more frequently showed an objective response (70/139; 50%) [60] than patients with ER-negative tumors (7%–33%) [37, 38]. In particular, Kaufmann et al. [38] reported an appreciable response rate in ER-poor patients (33%). They also found a high subjective response rate with improvement of the activity score in 51% and of the pain score in 78%. The median duration of response was in excess of 11 months in their study and in excess of 15 months in the study of Dixon et al. [37], with the longest duration in complete responders (9%–10%). Surgical

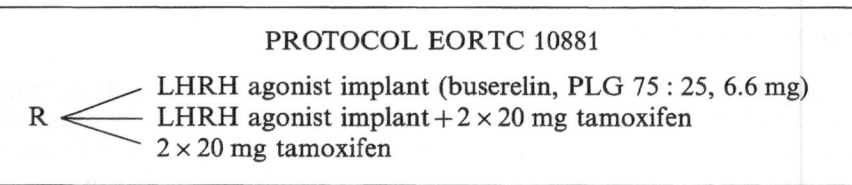

Fig. 2. Study design of a randomized study comparing combined treatment versus single treatment (EORTC 10881)

Table. 1. Antitumor effects in 46 premenopausal patients

Group	Treatment	CR+PR (n)	No change (n)	Failure (n)	n
I A	Buserelin intranasally	4	4	4	12
I B	Buserelin subcutaneously	5	1	5	11
II A	Buserelin intranasally + TAM	3	0	2	5
II B	Buserelin intranasally + MA	2	1	1	4
II C	Buserelin subcutaneously + TAM	4	3	7	14
Total		18 (39%)	9 (20%)	19 (41%)	46

CR, complete remission; PR, partial remission; TAM, tamoxifen; MA, megestrole acetate.

Table 2. Results of single LH-RH agonist treatment in premenopausal metastatic breast cancer

First author	LH-RH agonist	n	CR + PR	
			n	%
Klijn [21–24]	Buserelin	23	9	39
Nicholson [26]	Goserelin	45	14	31
Harvey [28]	Leuprolide	25	11	44
Mathé [30]	Triptorelin	8	3	38
Höffken [29]	Buserelin	19	8	42
Höffken [58]	Buserelin	12	4	33
Wander [55]	Goserelin	10	6	60
Kauffmann [56]	Goserelin	12	5	42
Kauffmann [38]	Goserelin	118	53	45
Bianco [57]	Goserelin	50	14	28
Nomura [59]	Goserelin	10	4	40
Dixon [37]	Goserelin	75	25	33
Dowsett [39]	Leuprolide	12	5	42
Total		419	161	39

CR, complete remission; PR, partial remission.

Table 3. Results of single LH-RH agonist therapy in postmenopausal metastatic breast cancer

First author	LH-RH agonist	n	CR + PR	
			n	%
Harvey [28]	Leuprolide	41[a]	4	10
Mathé [30]	Triptorelin	15[a]	3	20
Plowman [52]	Goserelin	10	2	20
Waxman [51]	Buserelin	18	0	0
Harris [48]	Goserelin	28[a]	3	11
Crighton [53]	Leuprolide	15[a]	0	0
Total		127	12	9

[a] Most of them pretreated with other agents.

oophorectomy after disease progression did not promote further tumor remissions in the great majority of a group of 45 patients [26].

Postmenopausal Patients

A few investigators studied the efficacy of LH-RH agonists in a total of 135 postmenopausal patients (Table 3) [28, 30, 48, 51–55]. The response rate reported varied between 0% and 20%, with an overall response rate of 9%.

Combination Treatments with LH-RH Agonists

Antiestrogens

In rats with DMBA-induced mammary tumors, the pure antiestrogen ICI 164-884 showed a greater antitumor effect in combination with the LH-RH agonist Zoladex than tamoxifen, probably due to the lack of weak estrogen agonistic properties observed for tamoxifen [35]. In clinical studies, mainly tamoxifen has been used in combination with LH-RH agonists. Tamoxifen stimulates pituitary-ovarian function, especially during the first period of chronic treatment [18, 45]. Very high plasma estradiol concentrations have been found in a significant number of patients, although amenorrhea may occur during prolonged treatment in some patients. In spite of the absence of "medical castration", tamoxifen causes a response rate similar to that for oophorectomy, i.e., approximately 30% in unselected premenopausal patients [40, 61–63] and acts by blocking the growth-stimulating effects of estradiol directly at the level of tumor cells. In analogy to the intended complete androgen blockade by combination therapy in patients with metastatic prostate cancer [64–66], "complete estrogen blockade" using LH-RH analogs in combination with antiestrogens may cause more rapid relief of complaints and hopefully an improvement in response rate, duration of response, and survival in patients with metastatic breast cancer. Our studies showed that subcutaneous administration of daily injections of buserelin [31] or 2-monthly implants [46] can safely be combined with tamoxifen in the presence of continuous suppression of pituitary-ovarian function. A potential disadvantage of this combination therapy might be (partial) abolishment of the direct inhibitory effect of LH-RH analogs on tumor cell growth, which may be caused by opposite effects on PgR synthesis, as demonstrated in our preclinical studies (Foekens and Klijn, this volume) [67]. On the other hand, we have observed objective tumor regression in 7 out of 19 patients treated with this drug combination. Patients with the combination treatment tended to have a somewhat better survival [24]. In a non-randomized comparative phase II study, Nicholson et al. [36] also found a longer survival in patients treated with Zoladex plus tamoxifen than in patients treated with Zoladex alone. Strikingly, a lower objective response rate, but a higher proportion of static disease, was observed with the combination of the drugs without a difference in the occurrence of progressive disease. They found no adverse endocrinological interaction between the drugs, but rather a more effective suppression of FSH secretion and slightly but significantly lower plasma estradiol levels during combination therapy [36]. In our experience, however, plasma estradiol levels are slightly but not significantly higher during combination therapy [31]. Remissions were primarily restricted to patients with ER-positive tumors [36]. Interestingly, patients with ER-negative tumors tended to respond less well to combination therapy [36]. In this respect, it is worthwhile to note that Szende et al. [68] reported an adverse effect of tamoxifen with LH-RH agonist on the growth of ER-negative MXT mouse mammary carcinoma. Presently, different large prospective randomized phase III trials are being conducted and these will still have to prove the possible superiority of combined versus single agent therapy.

Progestins and Antiprogestins

Previously we have treated a few patients with buserelin and megestrol acetate (160 mg per day) [18, 21]. Plasma gonadotropin and estradiol levels were clearly suppressed during combination therapy, but single treatment with high-dose progestins caused the same endocrine effects. Some long-term responders were observed.

The combination of buserelin and the antiprogestin mifepristone (RU 486) caused the highest tumor remissions in rats with DMBA-induced mammary tumors and was more effective than single treatment with various antihormonal agents [50].

Aromatase Inhibitors

In premenopausal women, LH-RH agonists suppress plasma estradiol levels to postmenopausal values. Aromatase inhibitors are known to decrease plasma estradiol levels by about 50% in postmenopausal women. Consequently an additive effect of combination treatment on plasma estradiol levels may be expected. Indeed, Stein et al. [69] showed that addition of 4-hydroxyandrostenedione (4OHA) to treatment with Zoladex led to a further suppression of estradiol (from 24 to 6 pmol/l) to within the range observed in postmenopausal patients treated with 4OHA. Whether these favorable endocrine effects will result in higher response rates has to be proven in randomized trials.

Somatostatin Analogs

In MXT mammary carcinoma, a combination of the somatostatin analog RC-160 and the LH-RH agonist Decapeptyl appeared slightly more effective than single therapy with each of these agents [70]. In rats with DMBA-induced mammary tumors we found no additive effect of Sandostatin (octreotide) when combined with buserelin, but single Sandostatin treatment appeared not effective in this model, probably as a consequence of a lack of somatostatin receptors in these tumors [71]. Clinical studies are presently awaited.

LH-RH Antagonists

LH-RH antagonists may offer certain advantages in the treatment of cancer as compared with superagonists [11, 16, 17]. The inhibition of gonadotropin release by LH-RH antagonists starts immediately after its administration, while the agonists cause a transient stimulation. Furthermore, antagonists may have a longer duration of action. On the other hand, LH-RH antagonists are more expensive and cause more side effects then agonists. So, it might be worthwhile to start treatment with an antagonist and then to continue with an agonist for long-term treatment. On the other hand, recently developed antagonists proved to have a greater antitumor potency than agonists and were even more effective than surgical castration in an experimental model [17]. In view of the fact that the newer LH-RH antagonists cause fewer side effects than the original ones [11, 17], chronic single treatment with an LH-RH antagonist might be also attractive.

Side Effects

No serious side effects occurred with the exception of those caused by the intended hypogonadism, i.e., hot flushes, decreased libido, and in a few patients mental depression [15]. Hot flushes were experienced as soon as plasma estradiol concentrations dropped to castration values. The frequency of the flushes varied between 3 and 30 times per day. During the years of treatment, the intensity decreased. A few patients treated with high-dose subcutaneous injections showed short-term (10–60 min) urticarial skin irritation at the injection site without pain or itching. However, as in other studies, we did not observe this type of side effect in patients ($n = 16$) treated with buserelin implants (for 3 to more than 24 months) [31–33, 46]. Initial tumor flare with LH-RH agonist treatment, as observed in a small percentage of prostate cancer patients due to early transient rises of steroids, has not been reported or well documented in any of the publications on advanced breast cancer [1].

Discussion

Treatment with medical castration using LH-RH analogs is quite a new approach in the treatment of hormone-dependent tumors. Using relatively low dosages, there is a great interindividual variation in endocrine response. While there is little difference in potency between the commonly used LH-RH analogs, some patients need 100 times higher dosages than others to reach medical castration levels. However, provided that sufficiently high subcutaneous dosages by injection (at least 1 mg/day) or by implants are used, medical castration will be reached in all patients [31–39]. Presently, mainly depot formulations are used in clinical practice. The decrease in plasma estradiol levels to castration values is slower (about 2–3 weeks) than observed after surgical castration (about 2–7 days) [34, 35]. This might be overcome by the temporary administration of LH-RH antagonists instead of agonists at the start of treatment [11]. Radiotherapeutical castration takes more time (about 6 weeks) before the optimal endocrine effect has been reached. The absence of side effects of LH-RH agonist treatment is an important advantage of this treatment modality.

In rats with DMBA-induced mammary tumors, we [72] and others [8] did not find a difference in antitumor efficacy between surgical castration and medical castration with LH-RH analog treatment. Based on noncomparative clinical studies, chronic LH-RH agonist treatment of premenopausal patients with advanced breast cancer appears as effective as common kinds of endocrine therapy, surgical or radiotherapeutic castration, or treatment with tamoxifen with respect to response rate, duration of response, and survival.

Randomized studies are presently being conducted to compare the efficacy of LH-RH agonist treatment with that of conventional treatment methods or of combined treatment modalities (Fig. 1) [73]. Slow-release depot formulations of LH-RH agonists, administered once every 4–12 weeks, are now commonly used in most trials and represent a comfortable mode of treatment for patients [33]. The reported 10% response rate in postmenopausal patients (Table 3) can be explained by indirect endocrine antitumor effects [1, 47, 48] apart from direct growth inhibitory effects [14] (Foekens and Klijn, this volume). Nevertheless, an additional advantage of the continuous release of LH-RH agonist by implants in the sense of direct growth inhibitory effects on human breast cancer cells remains possible.

Conclusions

1. In premenopausal metastatic breast cancer, chronic LH-RH agonist treatment appears as effective as other common kinds of endocrine therapy with respect to response rate, duration of response, and survival.
2. LH-RH agonist treatment with implants is the most effective and convenient way of treatment.
3. In aiming at "complete estrogen blockade", LH-RH agonist implants can be safely combined with tamoxifen. Combinations with other drugs might also be attractive.
4. No serious side effects have been observed.
5. The reported tumor remissions in some postmenopausal patients can be explained by both indirect endocrine antitumor and direct antitumor effects.

Future Prospects

For the future, the following questions remain to be answered and warrant clinical investigations

1. Controlled, randomized prospective studies to compare LH-RH agonists with ovariectomy or tamoxifen.
2. Administration of longer-acting sustained release preparations, which can be injected once every 3–6 months.

3. Use of LH-RH antagonists in clinical trials.
4. Use of LH-RH analogs in combination therapy aiming at more effective treatment modalities.
5. Use of LH-RH analogs in hormonal synchronization regimens before chemotherapy.
6. Use of LH-RH analogs in adjuvant therapy.
7. Use of LH-RH analogs in the prevention of breast cancer, maybe in combination with low-dose conjugated equine estrogens in order to prevent the potential increased risk of osteoporosis and coronary heart disease [74].

References

1. Santen RJ, Manni A, Harvey H, Redmond C (1990) Endocrine treatment of breast cancer in women. Endocr Rev 11: 221–265
2. Dowsett M (1990) Novel approaches for the endocrine therapy of breast cancer. Eur J Cancer 26: 989–992
3. Klijn JGM, de Jong FH (1982) Treatment with a luteinizing hormone-releasing-hormone analogue (Buserelin) in premenopausal patients with metastatic breast cancer. Lancet I: 1213–1216
4. Schally AV, Redding TW, Comaru-Schally AM (1984) Potential use of analogs of luteinizing hormone-releasing hormones in the treatment of hormone-sensitive neoplasms. Cancer Treat Rep 68: 281–289
5. Manni A, Santen R, Harvey H, Lipton A, Max D (1986) Treatment of breast cancer with gonadotropin releasing hormone. Endocr Rev 7: 89–94
6. Waxman J (1987) Gonadotrophin hormone releasing analogues open new doors in cancer treatment. Br Med J 295: 1084–1085
7. Corbin A (1982) From contraception to cancer: a review of the therapeutic applications of LH-RH analogues as antitumor agents. Yale J Biol Med 55: 27–47
8. Furr BJA, Nicholson RI (1982) Use of analogues of luteinizing hormone-releasing hormone for the treatment of cancer. J Reprod Fertil 64: 529–539
9. Sandow J (1983) Clinical applications of LH-RH and its analogues. Clin Endocrinol (Oxf) 18: 571–592
10. Schally AV, Srkalovic G, Szende B, Redding TW, Janaky T, Juhasz A, Korkut E, Cai RZ, Szepeshazik, Radulovic S, Bokser L, Groot K, Serfozo P, Comaru-Schally AM (1990) Antitumor effects of analogs of LH-RH and somatostatin: experimental and clinical studies. J Steroid Biochem Mol Biol 37: 1061–1069
11. Conn PM, Crowly WF (1991) Gonadotropin-releasing hormone and its analogues. N Engl J Med 324: 93–103
12. Desombre ER, Johnson ES, White WF (1976) Regression of rat mammary tumors effected by a gonadoliberin analog. Cancer Res 36: 3830–3833
13. Danguy A, Legros N, Heuson-Stiennon JA, Pasteels JL, Atassi G, Heuson JC (1977) Effects of a gonadotropin-releasing hormone (GnRH) analogue (A-43818) on 7,12-dimethylbenz(a)anthracene-induced rat mammary tumours. Histological and endocrine studies. Eur J Cancer 13: 1089–1094
14. Klijn JGM, Foekens JA (1989) Extrapituitary actions. In: Vickery BH, Lunenfeld B (eds) GnRH analogues in cancer and human reproduction: basic aspects, vol 1. Kluwer, Dordrecht, pp 71–85
15. Klijn JGM (1988) LH-RH agonists in the treatment of metastatic breast cancer: five years experience. In: Höffken K (ed) LH-RH Agonists in Oncology. Springer, Berlin Heidelberg New York, pp 139–147
16. Sharoni Y, Bosin E, Miinster A, Levy J, Schally AV (1989) Inhibition of growth of human mammary tumor cells by potent antagonists of luteinizing hormone-releasing hormone. Proc Natl Acad Sci USA 86: 1648–1651

17. Szende B, Srkalovic G, Groot K, Lapis K, Schally AV (1990) Growth inhibition of mouse MXT mammary tumor by the luteinizing hormone-releasing hormone antagonist SB-75. J Natl Cancer Inst 82: 513–517
18. Klijn JGM (1984) Long-term LH-RH-agonist treatment in metastatic breast cancer as a single treatment and in combination with other additive endocrine treatment. Med Oncol Tumor Pharmacother 1: 123–128
19. Klijn JGM, de Jong FH, Blankenstein MA, Docter R, Alexieva-Figusch J, Blonk-van der Wijst J, Lamberts SWJ (1984) Antitumor and endocrine effects of chronic LH-RH agonist (Buserelin) treatment with or without tamoxifen in premenopausal metastatic breast cancer. Breast Cancer Res Treat 4: 209–220
20. Klijn JGM, de Jong FH (1984) Long-term treatment with the LH-RH-agonist Buserelin (Hoe 766) for metastatic breast cancer in single and combined drug regimen. In: Labrie F, Belanger A, Dupont A (eds) LH-RH and its analogues, basic and clinical aspects. Excerpta Medica, Amsterdam, pp 425–437
21. Klijn JGM, de Jong FH, Lamberts SWJ, Blankenstein MA (1985) LH-RH-agonist treatment in clinical and experimental human breast cancer. J Steroid Biochem 23: 867–873
22. Klijn JGM, Henkelman MS, Bakker GH (1987) Treatment of premenopausal women with advanced breast cancer or endometriosis with LH-RH analogues. In: Engelsman E (ed) Proceedings of the symposium on endocrine-related tumours (May 1985, Noordwijkerhout). Update Siebert, Guildford, pp 160–169
23. Klijn JGM, de Jong FH (1987) Long-term LH-RH-agonist (Buserelin) treatment in metastatic premenopausal breast cancer. In: Klijn JGM, Paridaens R, Foekens JA (eds) Hormonal manipulation of cancer: peptides, growth factors and new (anti)steroidal agents. Raven, New York, pp 343–352 (EORTC Monograph Series, vol 18)
24. Klijn JGM, Foekens JA (1987) Long-term peptide hormone treatment with LH-RH agonists in metastatic breast cancer. In: Santen R, Juhos E (eds) Proceedings of the international symposium on endocrine-dependent breast cancer: critical assessment of recent advances. 14th International Cancer Congress, Budapest (23rd August 1986). Hans Huber, Bern, pp 92–102
25. Nicholson RI, Walker KJ, Turkes A, Dyas J, Plowman PN, Williams M, Blamey RW (1985) Endocrinological and clinical aspects of LH-RH action (ICI-118630) in hormone dependent breast cancer. J Steroid Biochem 23: 843–849
26. Nicholson RI, Walker KJ, Turkes A, Dyas J, Plowman PN, Williams M, Elston CW, Blamey RW (1987) The British experience with LH-RH agonist Zoladex (ICI-118630) in the treatment of breast cancer. In: Klijn JGM, Paridaens R, Foekens JA (eds) Hormonal manipulation of cancer: peptides, growth factors and new (anti)steroidal agents. Raven, New York, pp 331–343 (EORTC Monograph Series, vol 18)
27. Harvey HA, Lipton A, Max DT (1984) LH-RH-analogs for human mammary carcinoma. In: Vickery BH, Nestor JJ, Hafex ESE (eds) LH-RH and its analogues, contraceptive and clinical application. MTP Press, Lancaster, pp 329–338
28. Harvey HA, Lipton A, Max DT, Pearlman HG, Diaz-Perches R, de la Garza J (1985) Medical castration produced by the GnRH analogue Leuprolide to treat metastatic breast cancer. J Clin Oncol 3: 1068–1072
29. Höffken K, Miller B, Fischer P, Becker R, Kurschel E, Scheulen ME, Miller AA, Callies R, Schmidt CG (1986) Buserelin in treatment of premenopausal advanced breast cancer. Eur J Cancer Clin Oncol 22: 746
30. Mathé G, Keiling R, Vovan ML, Gastiaburu J, Prevot G, Vannetzel JM, Despax R, Jasmin C, Lévi F, Musset M, Machover D, Misset JL (1986) Phase II trial of D-Trp-6-LH-RH in advanced breast cancer. Eur J Cancer Clin Oncol 22: 723
31. Klijn JGM, van Geel AN, Sandow J, de Jong FH (1988) Treatment with high dose LH-RH agonist (buserelin) plus tamoxifen and with buserelin implants in premenopausal patients: an endocrine and pharmacokinetic study. In: Bresciani F, King RJB, Lippman ME, Raynaud JP (eds) Hormones and Cancer 3. Raven, New York, pp 365–368
32. Klijn JGM, van Geel AN, de Jong FH, Sandow J (1990) Endocrine, pharmacokinetic and clinical effects of LH-RH analogue treatment in patients with malignant and

benign breast disease. In: Vickery BH, Lunenfeld B (eds) GnRH analogues in cancer and human reproduction: benign and malignant tumours, vol 3. Kluwer, Dordrecht, pp 193–203

33. Klijn JGM, van Geel B, de Jong FH, Sandow J, Krauss B (1991) The relation between pharmacokinetics and endocrine effects of buserelin implants in patients with mastalgia. Clin Endocrinol 34: 253–258

34. Nicholson RI, Walker KJ (1989) Use of LH-RH agonists in the treatment of breast disease. In: Beck JS (ed) Oestrogen and the human breast. The Royal Society of Edinburgh, Edinburgh, pp 271–283

35. Nicholson RI, Walker KJ, Bouzubar N, Wills RJ, Gee JMW, Rushmere NK, Davies P (1990) Estrogen deprivation in breast cancer: clinical, experimental, and biological aspects. Ann New York Acad Sci 595: 316–327

36. Nicholson RI, Walker KJ, McClelland RA, Dixon A, Robertson JFR, Blamey RW (1990) Zoladex plus tamoxifen versus Zoladex alone in pre- and perimenopausal metastatic breast cancer. J Steroid Biochem Mol Biol 37: 989–997

37. Dixon AR, Robertson JFR, Jackson L, Nicholson RI, Walker KJ, Blamey RW (1990) Goserelin (Zoladex) in premenopausal advanced breast cancer: duration of response and survival. Br J Cancer 62: 868–870

38. Kaufmann M, Jonat W, Klieberg U, Eiermann W, Jänicke F, Hilfrich J, Kreienberg R, Albrecht M, Weitzel HK, Schmid H, Stunz P, Schachner-Wünschmann E, Bastert G, Maas H, German Zoladex Trial Group (1989) Goserelin, a depot gonadotrophin-releasing hormone agonist in the treatment of premenopausal patients with metastatic breast cancer. J Clin Oncol 7: 1113–1119

39. Dowsett M, Mehta A, Mansi J, Smith IE (1990) A dose-comparative endocrine-clinical study of leuprolin in premenopausal breast cancer patients. Br J Cancer 62: 834–837

40. Smith IE (1991) LH-RH analogues in breast cancer: clever, but do we need them? Br J Cancer 63: 15–16

41. Sandow J, Clayton RH (1983) The disposition, metabolism, kinetics and receptor binding properties of LH-RH and its analogues. In: Briggs M, Corbin A (eds) Progress in hormone-biochemistry and pharmacology, vol 2. Eden, Montreal, pp 63–106

42. Sandow J, Seidel HR, Krauss B, Jerabek-Sandow G (1987) Pharmacokinetic of LH-RH agonists in different delivery systems and the relation to endocrine function. In: Klijn JGM, Paridaens R, Foekens JA (eds) Hormonal manipulation of cancer: peptides, growth factors and new (anti)steroidal agents. Raven, New York, pp 203–212 (EORTC Monograph Series, vol. 18)

43. Sandow J, Fraser HM, Seidel H, Krauss B, Jerabek-Sandow G, von Rechenberg W (1987) Buserelin: pharmacokinetics, metabolism and mechanisms of action. Br J Clin Pract 41 [Suppl 48]: 6–13

44. Tharandt L, Schulte H, Benker G, Hackenberg K, Reinwein D (1979) Binding of luteinizing hormone-releasing hormone to human serum proteins – influence of a chronic treatment with a more potent analogue of LH-RH. Horm Metab Res 11: 391

45. Manni A, Pearson OH (1980) Antiestrogen-induced remissions in premenopausal women with stage IV breast cancer: effects on ovarian function. Cancer Treat Rep 64: 779–785

46. Klijn JGM, van Maarschalkerweerd MW, Sandow J, de Jong FH (1988) Treatment with LH-RH agonist (buserelin) implants once every 8 weeks in combination with tamoxifen for premenopausal metastatic breast cancer. Cancer Chemother Pharmacol 23 [Suppl. C47] (abstract 185)

47. Dowsett M, Cantwell B, Anshumala L, Jeffcoate SL, Harris AL (1988) Suppression of postmenopausal ovarian steroidogenesis with the luteinizing hormone-releasing hormone agonist goserelin. J Clin Endocrinol Metab 66: 672–677

48. Harris AL, Carmichael J, Cantwell BMJ, Dowsett M (1989) Zoladex: endocrine and therapeutic effects in postmenopausal breast cancer. Br J Cancer 59: 97–99

49. Williamson K, Robertson JFR, Ellis IO, Elston CW, Nicholson RI, Blamey RW (1988) Effect of LH-RH agonist Zoladex on ovarian histology. Br J Surg 75: 595–596

50. Bakker GH, Setyono-Han B, Portengen H, de Jong FH, Foekens JA, Klijn JGM (1989) Endocrine and antitumor effects of combined treatment with an antiprogestin and anti-estrogen or luteinizing hormone-releasing hormone agonist in female rats bearing mammary tumors. Endocrinology 125:1593–1598

51. Waxman JH, Harland SJ, Coombes RC, Wrigley PFM, Malpas JS, Powles T, Lister TA (1985) The treatment of postmenopausal women with advanced breast cancer with buserelin. Cancer Chemother Pharmacol 15:171–173

52. Plowman PN, Nicholson RI, Walker KJ (1986) Remissions of postmenopausal breast cancer during treatment with the luteinizing hormone-releasing hormone agonist ICI 118630. Br J Cancer 54:903–909

53. Crighton IL, Dowsett M, Lal A, Man A, Smith IE (1989) Use of luteinizing hormone-releasing hormone agonist (leuprorelin) in advanced postmenopausal breast cancer: clinical and endocrine effects. Br J Cancer 60:644–648

54. Schwartz L, Guiochet N, Keiling R (1988) Two partial remissions induced by an LH-RH analogue in two postmenopausal women with metastatic breast cancer. Cancer 62:2498–2500

55. Wander HE, Kleeberg UR, Schachner-Wünschmann E, Nagel GA (1987) A long-acting depot preparation of a synthetic GnRH agonist (Zoladex) in the treatment of pre- and postmenopausal advanced breast cancer. J Steroid Biochem 28 [Suppl. 104 S] (abstract C-017)

56. Kaufmann M (1987) Treatment of advanced breast cancer with a long-acting depot preparation of a synthetic GnRH-agonist (Zoladex) in premenopausal patients. Abstract book of the 4th EORTC breast cancer working conference. (Abstract F1.8)

57. Bianco AR, Calabresi F, Fiorentino M, Fosser V, Lenti R, Rosso R, Sismondi PG (1989) Gn-RH analogue goserelin (Zoladex) in the treatment of pre- and perimenopausal women with metastatic breast cancer. 5th European conference on clinical oncology (London, September 3–7)

58. Höffken K, Weinhardt O, Wandl U, Günzel K, Overkamp F, Scheulen ME, Calies R, Sandow J, Schmidt CG (1989) Depot buserelin in premenopausal breast cancer: a pharmacokinetic and endocrinological phase I–II study. 5th European conference on clinical oncology (London, September 3–7)

59. Nomura (1989) Zoladex in the treatment of breast cancer. International symposium on current controversies in breast cancer (Cambridge, September 8–9)

60. Klijn JGM (1991) Future trials of endocrine therapy in the management of advanced breast cancer. In: Howell A (ed) Current controversies in the treatment of cancer, vol. 1: the role of antihormones. Parthenon, Carnforth, pp 51–65

61. Planting AST, Alexieva-Figusch J, Blonk-van der Wijst J, van Putten WLJ (1985) Tamoxifen therapy in premenopausal women with metastatic breast cancer. Cancer Treat Rep 69:363–368

62. Buchanan RB, Blamey RW, Durrant KR, Howell A, Paterson AG, Preece PE, Smith DC, Williams CJ, Wilson RG (1986) A randomized comparison of tamoxifen with surgical oophorectomy in premenopausal patients with advanced breast cancer. J Clin Oncol 4:1326–1330

63. Ingle JN, Krook JE, Green SJ, Kubista TP, Everson LK, Ahmann DL, Chang MN, Bisel HF, Windschitl HE, Twito DI, Pfeifle DM (1986) Randomized trial of bilateral oophorectomy versus tamoxifen in premenopausal women with metastatic breast cancer. J Clin Oncol 4:178–185

64. Labrie F, Belanger A, Dupont A, Emond J, Lacoursiere Y, Monfette G (1984) Combined treatment with LH-RH agonist and pure antiandrogen in advanced carcinoma of prostate. Lancet II:1090

65. Klijn JGM, de Voogt HJ, Schröder FH, de Jong FH (1985) Combined treatment with Buserelin and cyproterone acetate in metastatic prostatic carcinoma. Lancet II:493

66. Schröder FH, Lock TMTW, Chadha DR, Debruyne FMJ, Karthaus HFM, de Jong FH, Klijn JGM, Matroos AW, de Voogt HJ (1987) Metastatic cancer of the prostate managed with buserelin plus cyproterone acetate. J Urol 137:912–919

67. Foekens JA, Henkelman MS, Fukkink JF, Blankenstein MA, Klijn JGM (1986) Combined effects of buserelin, estradiol and tamoxifen on the growth of MCF-7 human breast cancer cells in vitro. Biochem Biophys Res Commun 140: 550–556
68. Szende B, Schally AV, Srkalovic G, Comaru-Schally AM, Wittliff JL (1989) Adverse effect of tamoxifen with LHRH agonist on oestrogen-receptor-negative mammary carcinoma. Lancet II: 222–223
69. Stein RC, Dowsett M, Hedley A, Gazet JC, Ford HT, Coombes RC (1990) The clinical and endocrine effects of 4-hydroxyandrostenedione alone and in combination with goserelin in premenopausal women with advanced breast cancer. Br J Cancer 62: 679–683
70. Szende B, Lapis K, Redding TW, Srkalovic G, Schally AV (1989) Growth inhibition of MXT mammary carcinoma by enhancing programmed cell death (apoptosis) with analogs of LH-RH and somatostatin. Breast Cancer Res Treatm 4: 307–314
71. Bakker GH, Setyono-Han B, Foekens JA, Portengen H, van Putten WLJ, de Jong FH, Lamberts SWJ, Reubi JC, Klijn JGM (1990) The somatostatin analog Sandostatin (SMS 201-995) in treatment of DMBA-induced rat mammary tumors. Breast Cancer Res Treatm 17: 23–32
72. Bakker GH, Setyono-Han B, Henkelman MS, de Jong FH, Lamberts SWJ, van der Schoot P, Klijn JGM (1987) Comparison of the actions of the antiprogestin Mifepristone (RU486), the progestin megestrol acetate, the LHRH analog buserelin, and ovariectomy in treatment of rat mammary tumors. Cancer Treat Rep 71: 1021–1027
73. Klijn JGM, van Zijl J, Beex L, Mauriac L, Becquart D, Julien JP, Garcia-Conde J, Piccart M, Jassem J, Burghouts J, Namer M, Mignolet F, Sylvester R, EORTC Breast Cancer Coop Group (1991) LHRH agonist versus LHRH agonist plus tamoxifen versus tamoxifen alone in the treatment of premenopausal breast cancer: a randomized phase III study (EORTC 10881). 5th EORTC breast cancer working conference (Leuven, September 3–6)
74. Pike MC, Ross RK, Lobo RA, Key TJA, Potts M, Henderson BE (1989) LHRH agonist and the prevention of breast and ovarian cancer. Br J Cancr 60: 142–148

LH-RH Agonists in the Treatment of Premenopausal Patients with Advanced Breast Cancer

K. Höffken

Innere Klinik und Poliklinik (Tumorforschung), Universitätsklinikum Essen, Hufelandstraße 55, W-4300 Essen, FRG

Introduction

Ovarian ablation has a long-standing history in the treatment of metastatic breast cancer. At the end of the last century, Schinzinger [34] and Beatson [1] independently reported on the beneficial effect of surgical removal of the ovaries in premenopausal women with advanced breast cancer. Subsequently, this treatment became the standard systemic hormonal therapy in such patients.

Such therapy has drawbacks, however. First, as shown in a random premenopausal patient population, oophorectomy produces an average 33% objective response rate [3, 12, 15, 17, 24, 32]. Thus, this treatment has the disadvantage that only a minority of patients respond and the remainder suffer unnecessary treatment morbidity. Second, since its introduction, hormone receptor determinations have assisted in predicting hormonal therapy effectiveness. This has resulted in nearly 70% response rates in patients with hormone receptor positive tumors. However, there are still some patients who are oophorectomized unnecessarily (about one third) and some with receptor negative tumors who might respond to the hormonal ablation therapy (about one tenth).

For these reasons, less invasive methods of attaining a response to hormonal treatment in advanced breast cancer have been sought. Initially, this was attempted by treating premenopausal patients with high doses of an antiestrogen. Results of this approach, however, are still controversial both in terms of response rates and with regard to whether it is a reliable tool for predicting the effectiveness of subsequent ovarian ablation therapy [2, 15, 16, 17, 25, 26, 28, 30].

Soon after the introduction of luteinizing hormone releasing hormone (LH-RH) agonists designed for the treatment of primary sterility or endometriosis, it became apparent that – continuously administered – these substances induced a down-regulation of pituitary receptors thus leading to a sustained hypogonadotropic ovarian insufficiency [7, 33]. Subsequent preclinical studies showed that LH-RH agonists are effective in a variety of hormone dependent tumors, including DMBA-induced mammary tumors in female rats [27, 33].

During the past years, analogues of LH-RH have been investigated in pre- and postmenopausal women. Encouraging results have been obtained in premenopausal patients with metastatic breast cancer [8, 9, 13, 14, 18–23, 36]. In addition, endocrinological and pharmacokinetic studies have lead to the development of depot formulations allowing monthly or 2-monthly drug administrations. Here we report our experiences in using the LH-RH agonist buserelin in premenopausal advanced breast cancer.

Patients and Methods

Patients

Study I: Subcutaneous and Intranasal Administration. Twenty-four patients with histologically proven advanced breast cancer entered a phase II study of buserelin. Treatment was initiated with a 7-day loading course of 1 mg subcutaneously (s.c.) three times daily. Thereafter, patients received maintenance therapy either with 0.4 mg intranasally (i.n.) six times daily (12 patients) or with 0.3–1.0 mg s.c. two to three times daily (six patients). One patient received 2.4 mg i.n. throughout the treatment. In three patients, serum hormone analysis showed postmenopausal values resulting in their exclusion from evaluation. All evaluable patients were biochemically proven premenopausal and had measurable tumor parameters. In all patients, buserelin was the first systemic treatment except for adjuvant chemotherapy, which had been terminated at least 6 months previously. All patients exhibited unequivocal evidence of progressive metastatic disease before initiation of buserelin treatment. Except for irradiation of local metastases, no concomitant tumor-specific treatment was allowed. In cases requiring irradiation, the local responses were excluded from evaluation of the overall response.

Study II: Subcutaneous Depot Administration. Twelve patients with histologically proven advanced breast cancer entered a second phase II study on buserelin. Treatment consisted of 6.6 mg buserelin as a depot formulation embedded in a rod of polylactic-polyglykol polymer matrix given monthly (six patients; 50:50 copolymer) or every 8 weeks (six patients; 75:25 copolymer). Two patients were initially on intranasal buserelin treatment and changed to the depot treatment during stable responses. The remaining patients exhibited unequivocal evidence of progressive metastatic disease before initiation of buserelin treatment. Except for irradiation of local metastases, no concomitant tumor-specific treatment was allowed. In cases requiring irradiation, the local responses were excluded from evaluation of the overall response.

Response Criteria

Responses were assessed according to the UICC guidelines [11]. Complete remissions were defined as disappearance of all tumor lesions including tumor-related symptoms. Partial objective tumor remission was defined as either a 50% decrease in the sum of the products of all measurable lesions or a recalcification of lytic bone lesions but no development of new lesions. The stable disease category (no change) included patients with isolated bone lesions who did not show progression or new lesions and also had subjective relief of bone pain for at least 2 months. The progressive disease category included patients who developed new lesions or exhibited an increase in old lesions. Response duration was defined as the interval between first demonstration of complete remission or start of buserelin treatment (for partial remissions and stable diseases), respectively, and the first documentation of diseases progression.

Clinical Evalution and Hormone Assays

Case histories, physical and laboratory examinations including complete blood counts, serum electrolytes, as well as liver, renal, and endocrine function studies were performed weekly for the first 6 weeks of treatment and monthly thereafter. Using commercially available radioimmunoassays, serum levels of the following hormones were determined:estradiol, progesterone, luteinizing hormone, and follicle stimulating hormone.

Pharmacokinetics

In patients receiving depot buserelin, serum and urine samples were collected for determination of buserelin concentrations by a radioimmunoassay as described previously [31]. This method is specific for the agonist structure, but does not discriminate between the intact decapeptide and the inactive metabolites.

In Vitro Investigations

Cells of the breast cancer cell line MCF-7 were grown in RPMI supplemented with 10% FCS at 37 °C in humidified air containing 10% CO_2. Single cell suspensions were obtained by incubation with 0.25% trypsin for 15 min. After two washes in medium cells were grown in 0.3% semisolid agar in the presence of RPMI medium containing 20% FCS or increasing concentrations of buserelin diluted in the medium. Cultures were incubated at 37 °C in humidified air containing 10% CO_2. Cell colonies were counted after 12 days and results were expressed as the percentage clonogenicity (number of cells forming colonies) in relation to colony growth in medium controls.

Results

The major clinical characteristics of the 24 patients who entered the first trial are outlined in Table 1. While all the patients were evaluable for toxicity, only 21 patients (88%) met the criteria for response evaluation. In the remaining three patients aged 42, 46, and 48 years, serum analysis showed post-menopausal hormone values despite a history of menstruation within the last year. All patients had received adjuvant chemotherapy, none of them responded to buserelin treatment.

The median age of the 21 patients evaluated was 41 years, and the median Karnofsky performance status was 90%.

In more than half of the patients, the estrogen receptor status of primary or metastatic lesions was positive, and in a quater unknown, 19% of the patients had a negative hormone receptor status.

A notable predominance of locoregional metastatic lesions refractory to local surgery or irradiation was observed. Pleuropulmonal metastases occurred in 14% and bone metastases in 33% of the patients. In one patient both locoregional and pleuro-pulmonal metastases were observed.

The median interval between mastectomy and first appearance of metastatic disease was 14 months. None of the patients had been hormonally pretreated; 25% had received prior adjuvant chemotherapy which had been terminated more than 6 months previously.

Response to Therapy

Study I. Table 2 shows the overall responses to buserelin, including the 95% confidence intervals, of the 21 patients. Complete remissions lasting 6–32 + months were observed in 24% of the patients. Four of the five complete

Table 1. Characteristics of patients treated with subcutaneous and intranasal buserelin (study I)

Number of patients	24
Evaluable	21 (88%)
Median age (years) (range)	41 (30–49)
Median Karnofsky performance (%) (range)	90 (80–100)
Estrogen receptor status	
Positive	12 (57%)
Unknown	5 (24%)
Negative	4 (19%)
Sites of metastases	
Locoregional[a]	12 (57%)
Pleuropulmonal[a]	3 (14%)
Bone	7 (32%)

[a] Both sites in one patient.

Table 2. Response to buserelin treatment in 21 premenopausal patients with advanced breast cancer

Results	Patients			Duration of responses (months)	
	no.	%	95% CI[a]	Median	Range
Complete remission	5	24	10%–53%	13+	6–32+
Partial remission	4	19	7%–46%	4	4–20
Stable disease	5	24	10%–53%	10+	3–15+
Progressive disease	7	33	16%–66%	–	–

[a] 95% confidence interval, poisson distribution.

Table 3. Response to buserelin treatment in relation to receptor status, relapse-free interval, and sites of metastases in 21 premenopausal patients with advanced breast cancer

	Patient (n)	CR/PR		NC	PD
		(n)	(%)		
Estrogen receptor					
Positive	11	5/2	58	3	2
Unknown	5	0/2	40	2	1
Negative	4	–	–	–	4
Relapse-free interval					
<2 years	13	1/2	17	3	7
≥2 years	8	4/2	75	2	–
Sites of metastases					
Locoregional[a]	12	5/1	50	2	4
Pleuropulmonal[a]	3	1/0	33	1	1
Bone	6	0/3	43	2	2

[a] Both sites in one patient.

responders had only locoregional metastases. One patient had pleuropulmonal and locoregional metastases. All patients had estrogen receptor positive tumors, and all but one had had a relapse-free interval of more than 2 years (see Table 3).

Partial responses with a median duration of 4 months were observed in 19% of the patients. Five patients (24%) experienced a stabilisation of previously progressive disease for 3–15+ months. Thirty three percent of the patients failed to respond to buserelin.

In Table 3, responses to buserelin treatment are related to estrogen receptor status, to the relapse-free interval between the time of mastectomy and the first appearance of metastases, and to the sites of metastases. It can be seen that patients with positive estrogen receptors (> 10 fmol/mg cytosol protein) and those with a relapse-free interval of more than 2 years responded well to the treatment. Conversely, all patients with negative hormone receptors and 83% of those with a short interval between primary tumor and metastases did not respond objectively (complete or partial remissions) to the treatment with buserelin. Due to the small numbers no conclusions could be drawn with regard to the sites of metastases. Complete and partial remissions were achieved in locoregional as well as in pleuropulmonal and bone lesions. It should be noted, however, that complete remissions occurred mainly in locoregional metastases. There was no conclusive correlation between histology of the primary breast cancer or between the route of administering maintenance therapy (subcutaneous versus intranasal) and remission rates (data not shown).

Study II. Table 4 shows the results of the 12 patients treated with depot buserelin subcutaneously every 4 and 8 weeks, respectively. Two patients could not be evaluated because they were treated with monthly depot buserelin after intranasal maintenance treatment for stable responses, and similarly a third patient was treated with buserelin depot every 8 weeks after stable response during monthly depot buserelin. Given the small numbers, no differences in response rates or response durations could be determined. Therefore, depot buserelin appears to be no less effective than the conventionally scheduled drug (see above, study I).

Side Effects

Study I. All patients experienced amenorrhea and tolerable hot flushes. In two patients a local allergic reaction was observed during the first days of subcutaneous injection of buserelin, most likely caused by the solvent of the drug.

Study II. All patients experienced amenorrhea and tolerable hot flushes. Local reactions occurred in two patients, once as a postimplantation hematoma that

Table 4. Response to treatment with 6.6 mg depot-buserelin in 12 premenopausal patients with advanced breast cancer

Results	Monthly implantation of 6.6 mg 50:50 matrix[a]		2-Monthly implantation of 6.6 mg 75:25 matrix[a]	
	Patients (*n*)	Duration (months)	Patients (*n*)	Duration (months)
Complete remission	–		–	
Partial remission	2	9, 12	2	6, 12
Stable disease	2	10, 10	2	7, 9
Progressive disease	–		1	
Not evaluable[a]	2		1	

[a] See text.

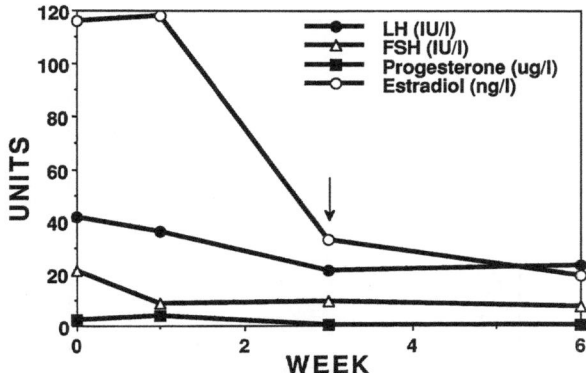

Fig. 1. Median serum hormone levels in premenopausal patients with advanced breast cancer before (week 0) and during treatment with subcutaneous and intranasal buserelin (study I)

resolved spontaneously, once as a minor inflammation that resolved under local antibiotics. In both patients, buserelin resorption was unchanged as evidenced by serum and urine buserelin levels as well as by the suppression of serum estradiol. The implanted rods could be palpated for approximately 8 weeks in the subcutaneous tissue.

Serum Hormone Levels

Study I. Figure 1 illustrates the changes in pituitary and ovarian hormone levels (median values) before (week 0) and during buserelin treatment. Castration levels of estradiol and progesterone were achieved 3 weeks after initiation of buserelin (arrow in Fig. 1). At the same time, LH decreased significantly and FSH remained in the range of pretherapeutic values in spite of the suppression of ovarian hormones.

Study II. Figure 2 illustrates the decrease in serum estradiol following the start of the depot buserelin treatment every 4 (Fig. 2a) or 8 (Fig. 2b) weeks. As can be seen, approximately 3 weeks after the onset of the treatment, postmenopausal estradiol levels were measured.

Pharmacokinetics

Buserelin excretion relative to renal function is shown in Fig. 3. For both administration schedules, urine concentration remained above the level of 1 µg/g creatinine. Here as in the serum estradiol levels, fluctuations were more pronounced when the drug was given every 8 weeks (Fig. 3b). However, the levels remained within the therapeutic range (above 1 µg buserelin per g crea-

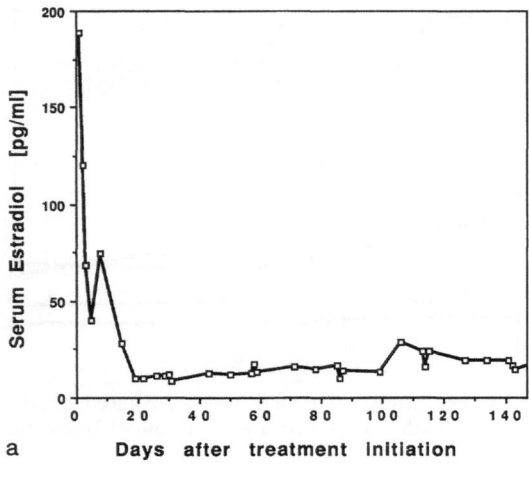

a

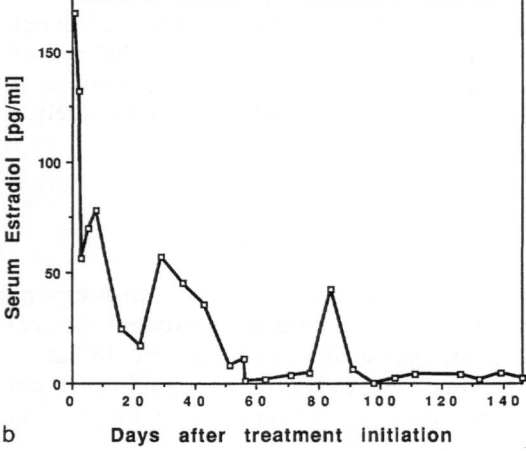

b

Fig. 2a, b. Median serum estradiol levels in premenopausal patients with advanced breast cancer before (day 0) and during treatment with 6.6 mg depot buserelin (study II) given every month (**a**) or every other month (**b**)

tinine). Buserelin serum levels after depot buserelin administration showed a similar pattern. As shown in Fig. 4 for the monthly treatment intervals, serum levels exhibited a relatively constant pattern of an initial increase immediately following depot implantation and a gradual decrease until the next implant.

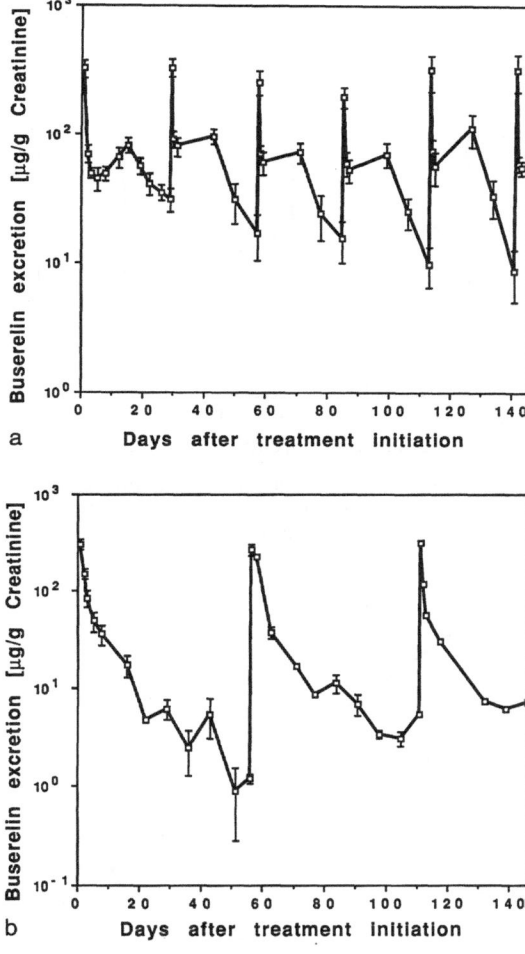

Fig. 3a, b. Mean (±SEM) urinary buserelin excretion (expressed in relation to creatinine excretion) in premenopausal patients with advanced breast cancer before (day 0) and during treatment with 6.6 mg depot buserelin (study II) given every month (**a**) or every other month (**b**)

In Vitro Investigations

Buserelin may inhibit breast cancer cell growth by mechanism(s) other than hormonal suppression. This direct antiproliferative effect-partly mediated by cellular LH-RH binding sites [4] – is demonstrated in Fig. 5. It is of note that the buserelin concentration necessary to suppress MCF-7 cell growth to 40% of the control is high, and would be reached in the serum of patients only by giving a dose some 10000-fold higher than that used to suppress ovarian estradiol production.

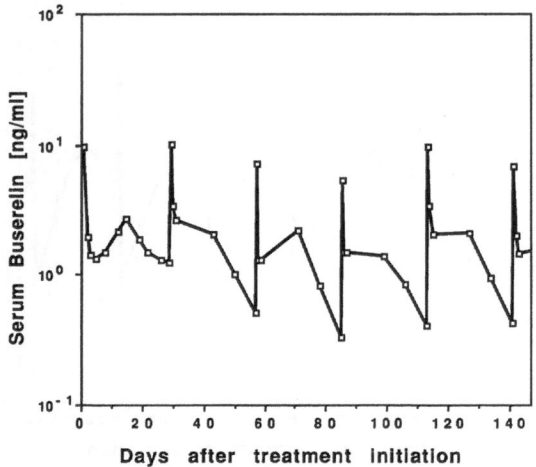

Fig. 4. Mean serum buserelin levels in premenopausal patients with advanced breast cancer before (day 0) and during treatment with 6.6 mg depot buserelin (50:50 copolymer matrix) (study II) given every month

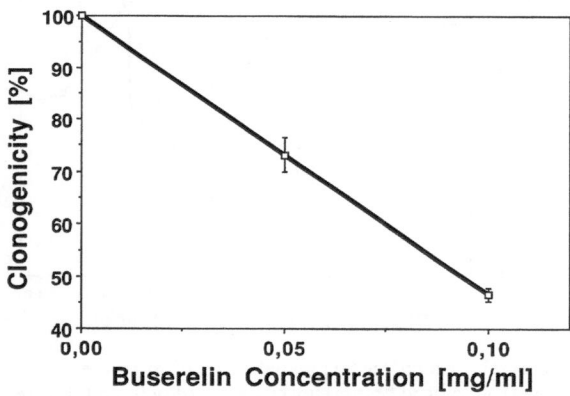

Fig. 5. Mean ($\pm$SEM) clonogenicity of MCF-7 breast cancer cells in vitro following exposure to increasing concentrations of buserelin as compared to medium control (0 mg/ml)

Discussion

The present study has shown that buserelin given subcutaneously and intranasally (study I) is effective in treating premenopausal patients with advanced breast cancer. The 43% objective remission rate observed here compares well with that of others using LH-RH agonists in this clinical setting [8, 9, 18–23, 36]. The relatively high complete remission rate achieved in the present study may be explained by the fact that it occurred in patients exhibiting mainly locoregional recurrences in conjunction with receptor positive tumors. However, pleuropulmonal and bone metastases also responded to buserelin treatment in 33% and 43%, respectively. It should be noted that all patients with receptor negative tumors and the majority of those who had had a short relapse-free interval failed to benefit from this hormonal ablation treatment. This is in accordance with the findings of Williams et al. [36], who did not see a single objective response in 18 patients with receptor negative tumors. Klijn et al. [20, 22, 23], however, achieved one remission out of two receptor negative patients, thus confirming the fact that due to a variety of reasons (e.g., handling of tumor specimen prior to receptor analysis, emergence of receptor positive metastases from apparently negative but heterogeneous primary tumors) the receptor negativity does not necessarily preclude a response to hormonal treatment of metastases.

In view of the response rates and response durations observed in this trial and by others using ovarian ablation therapy by LH-RH agonists it is tempting to speculate that "chemical castration" by these substances may replace oophorectomy. A note of caution is necessary, however, since Williams et al. [36] observed four patients who responded to surgical castration but failed to respond to prior LH-RH analog treatment. This question has obviously not yet been addressed systematically enough to allow a definite answer to be given. Moreover, the traditional approach to treat premenopausal patients with advanced breast cancer has been to irreversibly eliminate ovarian function so that after a transient remission other means of hormonal treatment (e.g., anti-estrogens, aromatase inhibitors) are faced with only minimal residual hormone activity such as estrogens produced by aromatization of adrenal androgens. Therefore, it still remains to be shown whether or not LH-RH agonist treatment has to provide a hormonal environment for the efficacy of subsequent hormone therapy. This would result in the requirement for either continuous treatment with LH-RH agonists even after termination of the remission or for surgical or radiotherapeutic ovarian ablation before initiation of a second hormonal therapy. Moreover, even with primary failure to oophorectomy subsequent hormone manipulations may be of benefit, thus asking for definite ovarian suppression also in these patients. The above questions are currently under investigation in several studies.

On the other hand, there is good evidence that LH-RH agonists directly inhibit tumor cell growth ([4, 5, 6, 33], Höffken unpublished findings, see Fig. 5). This is supported by case reports on the efficacy of these drugs in postmenopausal women [10, 29]. However, neither Waxman et al. [35] nor we observed an objective remission in such patients. In all three patients retrospectively proven by hormone profiles to be postmenopausal and therefore excluded from the analysis, disease progression occurred (data not shown). These patients were 42, 46, and 48 years of age; one had a receptor positive tumor and two a receptor unknown primary tumor; they had relapse-free intervals of 8, 12, and 48 months; the first two patients exhibited bone metastases and the third one lung metastasis. Interestingly, all patients had had adjuvant chemotherapy possibly leading to ovarian insufficiency.

With regard to the hormonal changes induced by the treatment with LH-RH agonists, the majority of patients reached castration levels after 3 weeks of therapy (Fig. 1). No attempt has been made to correlate the hormonal changes with the phase of the menstrual cycle in which buserelin therapy was started.

In a second study, we investigated the endocrine and clinical efficacy of a depot preparation of buserelin transplanted subcutaneously every 4 and 8 weeks, respectively. This drug formulation led to serum buserelin levels and urine excretion profiles sufficient to induce and maintain an estradiol suppression to postmenopausal values. In addition, clinical efficacy in the six patients treated by these regimens did not differ from that observed with the conventional sc/in route of administration. Thus, it appears that depot formulations given up to every 8 weeks are a safe way to induce ovarian failure for treatment of premenopausal patients with advanced breast cancer. This is in accordance with the findings of Kaufmann et al. [18].

Finally, in vitro studies using the MCF-7 breast cancer cell line confirmed a direct antiproliferative effect of buserelin on breast cancer cells, probably via cellular LH-RH binding sites [4]. The amount of drug necessary to show growth inhibition under these conditions, however, is some 10 000-fold higher than the serum levels reached by conventional dose buserelin treatment for premenopausal breast cancer patients.

In conclusion, LH-RH agonist treatment of premenopausal patients with advanced breast cancer appears to be effective with response rates and remission durations that are similar to that of oophorectomy. For this purpose, subcutaneous and intranasal applications are equivalent to depot preparations, the latter being superior in handling.

It remains to be determined, however, whether "chemical castration" can replace oophorectomy, especially with regard to a conceivably additional effect on the proliferative capacity of the tumor cell. Moreover, it has to be clarified whether buserelin efficacy, together with the hormone receptor status, can be used to predict a response to surgical ablation. Finally, combination of LH-RH agonists with other hormonal treatment strategies with different mechanisms of action are being explored.

Acknowledgements. The author gratefully acknowledges the cooperation of the following colleagues: C. U. Anders, R. Becher, R. Callies, E. Kurschel, C. Oesterdickhoff, M. E. Scheulen, and C. G. Schmidt. Dr. J. Sandow from Hoechst-Werke, Frankfurt-Main, FRG, performed the pharmacokinetic analyses in serum and urine samples mentioned in this paper. Mrs. F. Bosse is thanked for experimental, Mrs. G. Cönenberg for secreterial, and Mrs. R. Mühlich for data handling assistance. Behring-Werke AG, Marburg, FRG, provided us with buserelin.

References

1. Beatson GT (1896) On the treatment in operablic cases of carcinoma of the mamma: suggestions for a new method of treatment with illustrative cases Lancet 2:104–107, 162–165
2. Buchanan RB, Blamey RW, Durrant KR, Howell A, Paterson AG, Preece PE, Smith DC, Williams CJ, Wilson RG (1986) A randomized comparison of tamoxifen with surgical oophorectomy in premenopausal patients with advanced breast cancer. J Clin Oncol 4:1326–1330
3. Conte CC, Nemoto T, Rosner D, Dao TL (1989) Therapeutic oophorectomy in metastatic breast cancer. Cancer 64:150–153
4. Eidne KA, Flanagan CA, Harris NS, Millar RP (1987) Gonadotropin-releasing hormone (GnRH)-binding sites in human breast cancer cell lines and inhibitory effects of GnRH antagonists. J Clin Endocrinol Metab 64:425–32
5. Foekens JA, Henkelman MS, Bolt-deVries J, Portengen H, Fukkink JF, Blankenstein MA, van Steenbrugge GJ, Mulder E, Klijn JGM (1987) Direct effects of LHRH analogs on breast and prostatic tumor cells. In: Klijn JGM, Paridaens R, Foekens JA (eds) Hormonal manipulation of cancer: peptides, growth factor, and new (anti) steroidal agents. Monograph Series of the European Organization for Research on Treatment of Cancer (EORTC) 18:369–380
6. Foekens JA, Henkelman MS, Fukkink JF, Blankenstein MA, Klijn JGM (1986) Direct effects of LHRH analogs on tumor cells. Eur J Cancer 22:(Abstr III–s), 725
7. Hardt W, Schmidt GM (1983) Sustained gonadal suppression in fertile women with the LHRH agonist buserelin. Clin Endocrinol Oxf 19:613–7
8. Harvey HA, Lipton A, Max DT, Pearlman OHG, Diaz-Perches R, de la Garza J (1984) Effective medical castration produced by the GnRH analog Leuprolide in metastatic breast cancer. Proc Amer Soc Clin Oncol 3:(Abstr C-435), 111
9. Harvey HA, Lipton A, Max DT, Perlman OHG, Diaz-Perches R, de la Garza J (1985) Medical castration produced by the GnRH analog leuprolide to treat metastatic breast cancer. J Clin Oncol 3:1086–1072
10. Harvey HA, Lipton A, Santen RJ, Escher GC, Hardy MA, Glode LM, Sealoff A, Landau RL, Schneir H, Max DT (1981) Phase II study of a gonadotropin-releasing hormone analogue (Leuprolide) in postmenopausal advanced breast cancer patients. Proc Am Assoc Cancer Res & Amer Soc Clin Oncol 22:(Abstr C-436), 444
11. Hayward HA, Carbone PP, Heuson JC, Kumaoka S, Segaloff A, Rubens RD (1977) Assessment of response to therapy in advanced breast cancer. Eur J Cancer 13:89–94
12. Henderson IC, Cannelos GP (1980) Cancer of the breast: the past decade. N Engl J Med 302:17–30, 78–90
13. Höffken K (1988) LH-RH agonists in oncology. Springer, Berlin Heidelberg New York
14. Höffken K, Oesterdickhoff C, Becher R, Callies R, Kurschel E, Anders CU, Scheulen ME, Schmidt CG (1989) LH-RH agonist treatment with buserelin in premenopausal patients with advanced breast cancer: a phase II study. Cancer Ther Control 1:13–20
15. Hoogstraten B, Fletcher WS, Gad-el-Mawla N, Maloney TR, Altman SJ, Vaughn CB, Foulkes MA (1982) Tamoxifen and oophorectomy in the treatment of recurrent breast cancer. A southwest oncology group study. Cancer Res 42:4788–4791
16. Hoogstraten B, Gad-el-Mawla N, Maloney TR, Fletcher WS, Vaughn CB, Tranum BL, Athens JW, Costanzi JJ, Foulkes M (1984) Combined modality therapy for first recurrence of breast cancer. A Southwest Oncology Group Study. Cancer 54:2248–2256
17. Ingle JN, Krook JE, Green SJ, Kubista TP, Everson LK, Ahmann DL, Chang MN, Bisel HF, Windschitl HE, Twito DI, Pfeifle DM (1986) Randomized trial of bilateral oophrectomy versus tamoxifen in premenopausal women with metastatic breast cancer. J Clin Oncol 4:178–185
18. Kaufmann M, Jonat W, Kleeberg U, Eiermann W, Jänicke F, Hilfrich J, Kreienberg R, Albrecht M, Weitzel HK, Schmid H, Strunz P, Schachner-Wünschmann E, Bastert G, Maass H (1989) Goserelin, a depot gonadotropin-releasing hormone agonist in the

treatment of premenopausal patients with metastatic breast cancer. J Clin Oncol 7:1113–1119

19. Klijn JGM (1984) Long-term LHRH-agonist treatment in metastatic breast cancer as a single treatment and in combination with other additive endocrine treatments. Med Oncol Tumor Pharmacother 1:123–8

20. Klijn JGM, deJong FH (1982) Treatment with a luteinizing hormone-releasing hormone analogue ·(buserelin) in premenopausal patients with metastatic breast cancer. Lancet 1:1213–1216

21. Klijn JGM, deJong FH (1987) Long-term LHRH-agonist (Buserelin) treatment in metastatic premenopausal breast cancer. In: Klijn JGM, Paridaens R, Foekens JA (eds) Hormonal manipulation of cancer: peptides, growth factors, and new (anti) steroidal agents. Monograph Series of the European Organization for Research on Treatment of Cancer (EORTC) 18:343–352

22. Klijn JGM, deJong FH, Lamberts SWJ, Blankenstein MA (1985) LHRH-agonist treatment in clinical and experimental human breast cancer. J Steroid Biochem 23:867–873

23. Klijn JGM, Paridaens R, Foekens JA (1987) Hormonal manipulation of cancer: peptides, growth factors, and new (anti) steroidal agents. Monograph Series of the European Organization for Research on Treatment of Cancer (EORTC) 18:

24. Legha SS, Davis HL, Muggia FM (1978) Hormonal therapy of breast cancer: new approaches and concepts. Ann Intern Med 88:69–77

25. Manni A, Pearson OH (1976) Antiestrogen-induced remissions in stage IV breast cancer. Cancer Treat Rep 60:1445–1450

26. Manni A, Pearson OH (1980) Antiestrogen-induced remission in premenopausal women with stage IV breast cancer: effects on ovarian function. Cancer Treat Rep 64:779–785

27. Nicholson RI, Maynard PV (1979) Anti-tumour activity of ICI 118630, a new potent luteinizing hormone-releasing hormone agonist. Br J Cancer 39:268–273

28. Planting AST, Alexieva-Figusch J, Blonk-vdWist J, vanPutten WLJ (1985) Tamoxifen therapy in premenopausal women with metastatic breast cancer. Cancer Treat Rep 69:363–368

29. Plowman PN, Nicholson RI, Walker KJ (1986) Remissions of metastatic breast cancer in postmenopausal women with luteinizing hormone releasing hormone (ICI 118630) therapy. Eur J Cancer 22:746 (Abstract III-18)

30. Pritchard KI, Thomson DB, Myers RE, Sutherland D, Mobb BG, Meakin JW (1980) Tamoxifen therapy in premenopausal patients with metastatic breast cancer. Cancer Treat Rep 64:787–796

31. Sandow J, Fraser HM, Seidel H, Krauss B, Jarabek-Sandow G, Von Rechenberg W (1987) Buserelin: pharmacokinetics, metabolism and mechanisms of action. Br J Clin Pract 41:6–13

32. Schacter LP, Rozencweig M, Canetta R, Kelley S, Nicaise C, Smaldone L (1990) Overview of hormonal therapy in advanced breast cancer. Semin Oncol 17:38–46

33. Schally AV, Redding TW, Comaru SA (1984) Potential use of analogs of luteinizing hormone-releasing hormones in the treatment of hormone-sensitive neoplasms. Cancer Treat Rep 68:281–289

34. Schinzinger AS (1889) Über Carcinoma mammae. Zbl Chir (Beil) 16:55–56

35. Waxman JH, Harland SJ, Coombes RC, Wrigley P, Malpas JS, Powles T, Lister TA (1985) The treatment of postmenopausal women with advanced breast cancer with buserelin. Cancer Chemother Pharmacol 15:171–173

36. Williams MR, Walker KJ, Turkes A, Blamey RW, Nicholson RI (1986) The use of an LH-RH agonist (ICI 118630, Zoladex) in advanced premenopausal breast cancer. Br J Cancer 53:629–636

LH-RH Agonists in the Treatment of Pancreatic Cancer

D. Gonzalez-Barcena

Departamento Clinico de Endocrinologia, Hospital de Especialidades Centro Médico La Raza, Instituto Mexicano del Seguro Social, Seris y Zaachila, Col. La Raza, Mexico City, C.P. 02990, Mexico

Introduction

The incidence of adenocarcinoma of the exocrine pancreas is steadily increasing. Approximately 25 000 new cases of pancreatic cancer are diagnosed yearly in the United States where this tumor now ranks as the fourth leading cause of death from malignancies (Connolly et al. 1987; Greenberger et al. 1987). The vast majority of pancreatic cancers are ductal adenocarcinomas, but other pancreatic carcinomas also occur. Histogenetically, more than 90% of these tumors are derived from the pancreatic ducts and thus about 60% are located in the head of the gland (Moossa et al. 1986). Ductal adenocarcinoma has a very poor prognosis, in part because most patients have advanced disease by the time of diagnosis. Early diagnosis and screening for nonendocrine pancreatic cancer is difficult, although the technology for detecting these small tumors is available (Blind and Dahlgren 1987; Douglass 1987; Anonymous 1986; Malt 1983).

The majority of pancreatic carcinomas are diagnosed in advanced stages, and current methods of treatment are usually ineffective. Surgery seems to be the only modality with curative potential, but the resectability rate in most trials is only about 15% – 20% (Greenberger et al. 1987), and radiotherapy and chemotherapy are usually ineffective (Connolly et al. 1987; Kalser and Ellenberg 1985; Malt 1983; Skibber et al. 1985). Attempts have been made to increase the duration of postresection survival by combining radiotherapy with chemotherapy. Among the chemotherapeutic agents that have been investigated are 5-fluorouracil, streptozotocin, adriamycin, and mitomycin C (Connolly et al. 1987; Kalser and Ellenberg 1985). Long-term survival in histologically confirmed pancreatic carcinoma is a rare event (Connolly et al. 1987). Theve et al. (1983) reported that the median duration of survival of 629 patients with pancreatic cancer diagnosed in Sweden during the period 1966 – 1979 was only 2.5 months, and in the United States, Pollard reported a median survival of 2.3 months in 415 patients (Pollard et al. 1981).

Recent Results in Cancer Research, Vol. 124
© Springer-Verlag Berlin · Heidelberg 1992

The presence of specific receptors for estrogen and androgen in pancreatic carcinoma tissue indicates that sex hormones might influence neoplastic cell processes (Benz et al. 1986; Corbishley et al. 1986; Pousette et al. 1982; Theve et al. 1983). Both androgen and estrogen receptors were detected in human pancreatic adenocarcinoma and cancer cell lines. Confirmatory evidence that pancreatic adenocarcinoma might be sex-steroid dependent was obtained by the demonstration that testosterone stimulated the growth of xenografts of human pancreatic adenocarcinomas in nude mice (Greenway et al. 1982). Moreover, the receptors for the D-Trp^6 analog of luteinizing hormone releasing hormone ([D-Trp^6]-LH-RH) have been detected in hamster and human pancreatic cancer (Fekete et al. 1989). Recent findings indicate that [D-Trp^6]-LH-RH also directly inhibits the growth of the human pancreatic cancer cell line MIA PaCa-2 in vitro (Hierowski et al. 1985). These findings reinforce the concept that carcinomas of the exocrine pancreas seem to be sex-hormone sensitive (Camaru-Schally et al. 1988).

Patients and Methods

Inhibition of the growth of pancreatic acinar and ductal cancers in rat and hamster models by analogs of LH-RH and somatostatin was shown by Redding and Schally (1984). In 1986, we reported preliminary results on the use of the agonist [D-Trp^6]-LH-RH in the treatment of five patients with advanced adenocarcinoma of the pancreas (Gonzalez-Barcera et al. 1986). In view of the encouraging results, we decided in collaboration with Dr. A. V. Schally and R. A. M. Comaru Schally to continue the trials with [D-Trp^6]-LH-RH in 24 patients with unresectable adenocarcinoma and biopsy-proven adenocarcinoma of the pancreas. None of the patients had previously been treated and all had stage IV disease according to the classification of Pollard et al. (1981). A gastrointestinal and biliary bypass was performed in the majority of the patients. The median age at diagnosis was 60 ± 12.3 years, with a range of 33–82 years. Thirteen patients were male and 11 female. Patients included in these protocol were severely debilitated from advanced metastases and weight loss. Patients such as these, with poor performance status or jaundice from hepatic metastases, are not suitable candidates for intensive chemotherapeutic regimens.

The patients were admitted to the Endocrinology Department of the Hospital de Especialidades of the Medical Center La Raza, IMSS in Mexico City. Informed consent was obtained from all the patients after the therapeutic options available had been explained. The study was approved by the Scientific Research Committee of the Mexican Institute of Social Security (Protocol No. 2561-84-0036). In order to evaluate safety and efficacy before treatment, the following tests were performed on each patient: radioisotope bone, brain, and liver scans; chest X-ray and bone survey; full blood count; and serum determinations of creatinine, blood urea nitrogen (BUN), uric acid, bilirubin (total and direct), glucose, total protein, albumin, globulin, serum glutamic-oxaloacetic transaminase (SGOT), serum glutamic-pyruvic transaminase (SGPT), alkaline phosphatase, acide phosphatase, and sodium, potassium, chloride, bicarbonate, calcium, phosphate, and magnesium levels. In addition, urinalysis, urine culture, and electrocardiography were performed and 24-h urine calcium, phosphate, and creatinine clearance tested.

The LH-RH agonist [D-Trp^6]-LH-RH, which has the amino acid sequence (pyro)Glu-His-Trp-Ser-Tyr-D-Trp-Leu-Arg-Pro-Gly-NH$_2$, was generously supplied in the form of Decapeptyl (triptorelin) by Debiopharm SA, Lausanne, Switzerland. Therapy with [D-Trp^6]-LH-RH was started 3–31 days after by-pass surgery (in the first year the average was 16 days, but in the following years it was reduced to 3.1 days), at a dose of 1 mg/day subcutaneously for the first 7 weeks. Subsequently, the dose was reduced to 100 µg/day. These doses were chosen on the basis of our previous extensive clinical studies on prostate cancer.

Results

The initial administration of 1 mg [D-Trp^6]-LH-RH caused a marked elevation of luteinizing hormone (LH) and folicle-stimulating hormone (FSH), which lasted more than 24 h. However, 1 week later and throughout the therapy, the basal values of LH and FSH were below the normal range, and no increase in serum gonadotropin levels was obtained after administration of the analog (Fig. 1). Initial plasma estradiol in premenopausal women during treatment with [D-Trp^6]-LH-RH fell to castration levels and levels did not increase again during the time of therapy (Fig. 2).

Figure 3 shows the survival time of 24 patients. In seven of them, it was less than 4 months (± 1.9 months) and in 17, more than 4 months (± 7.46 months).

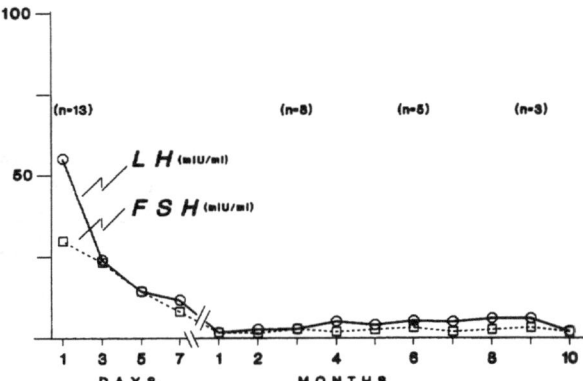

Fig. 1. Maximal serum luteinizing hormone (*LH*) and follicle-stimulating hormone (*FSH*) levels in patients with advanced pancreatic cancer (stage IV) during the subcutaneous administration of 100 µg/day [D-Trp^6]-LH-RH on the 1st, 3rd, 5th, and 7th day, and then once every month

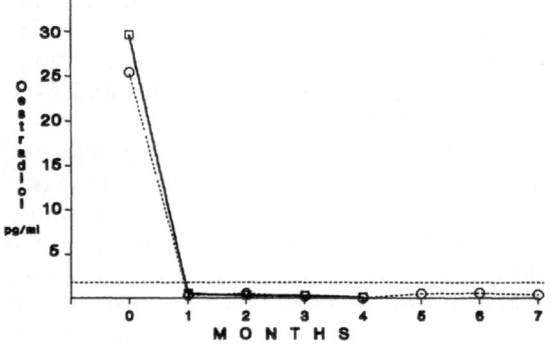

Fig. 2. Changes in serum estradiol in two premenopausal patients with advanced pancreatic cancer (stage IV) during therapy with 100 µg/day [D-Trp^6]-LH-RH administered subcutaneously

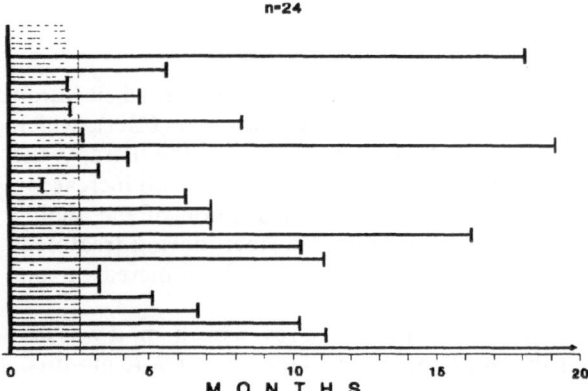

Fig. 3. Survival time of 24 patients with advanced pancreatic cancer treated with [D-Trp^6]-LH-RH. The *shaded area* represents the median duration of survival following conventional treatment modalities

After 3 weeks of [D-Trp^6]-LH-RH administration, we observed a subjective improvement in the patients, including a decrease in abdominal pain, reduction in serum bilirubin levels, und an increase in appetite and hemoglobin values. This improvement in the quality of life persisted until clinical relapse occurred about 2 weeks before death. In all cases a persistent blockade of the pituitary-gonadal-axis was obtained, producing a state of gonadal suppression, so-called chemical or medical castration (Gonzalez-Barcena et al. 1989).

Discussion

The relapse of the disease in spite of the medical castration obtained with the analog in all patients suggests that other factors are present. Regulation of growth of the exocrine pancreas appears to be hormonal in nature. The gastrointestinal hormones cholecystokinin (CCK) and secretin are the chief endocrine stimulants of pancreatic exocrine secretions. One important action of CCK, secretin, and gastrin that has recently been established is their ability to stimulate the growth of the exocrine pancreas. The role that these gastrointestinal hormones play in the development and growth of pancreatic cancer is not clearly understood, but it is likely that they may influence the growth of malignant cells of the pancreas.

A possible new approach to treat this malignancy has been proposed by our group (Gonzalez-Barcena et al. 1986, 1989; Redding and Schally 1984; Schally and Redding 1987; Schally et al. 1984; Szende et al. 1990), and is based on chronic administration of hormonal peptide analogs. The inhibitory effect of the LH-RH agonist [D-Trp[6]]-LH-RH and the somatostatin analog RC-160 on various experimental animal tumors including ductal pancreatic cancers has been demonstrated by our group (Szende et al. 1990). Various experimental and clinical findings suggest that it might be possible to develop a new hormonal therapy for malignant exocrine tumors of the pancreas based on new somatostatin analogs, alone or in combination with LH-RH. Potent analogs of somatostatin were synthesized by several groups including ours (Bauer et al. 1982; Cai et al. 1986, 1987).

Further Studies

Studies carried out during the past 14 years in several species, including human beings, have shown that somatostatin-14, somatostatin-28, and their analogs exert inhibitory actions on the endocrine and exocrine pancreas as well as on the stomach and gut (Konturek et al. 1976). These actions include inhibition of the release of insulin and glucagon from the pancreas and suppression of the secretion and/or action of gastrin, secretin, vasoactive intestinal peptide, and pancreatic polypeptide. Gastrin, CCK, cerulein, and secretin promote the growth of the exocrine pancreas and increase DNA, RNA, and protein content. The production of hyperplasia and hypertrophy of the exocrine pancreas by gastrin, CCK, and secretin is now well established. It is likely that these gastrointestinal hormones also influence the growth of the malignant cells of the pancreas and phenotypic transformations (Dembinski and Johnson 1980; Johnson 1981).

Recent evidence indicates that growth factors play an important role in pancreatic cancer. The fall in growth hormone (GH) levels induced by somatostatin analogs could be important for the inhibition of pancreatic tumor growth. GH stimulates local production of insulin-like growth factor 1 (IGF-1). IGF polypeptides, also called somatomedins, and various growth factors including epidermal growth factor (EGF), platelet-derived growth factor (PDGF), and transforming growth factor (TGF) appear to be involved in the proliferation of both normal and neoplastic cells or phenotypic transformation of cells (Goustin et al. 1986; Schally and Redding 1987). The human pancreatic cancer cell lines PANC-1 and MIA PaCa-2 have receptors for EGF. EGF stimulates the growth of MIA PaCa-2 pancreatic cancer cells in culture and may act as an autocrine growth factor (Kore and Magun 1985; Setyono et al. 1987). EGF also augments pancreatic carcinogenesis induced by bisoxopropyl (BOP) (Chester et al. 1986). Somatostatin reduces the levels of IGF-1 and EGF (Schally and Redding 1987), and nullifies cell replication in HeLa cells and growth of MIA PaCa-2 cells induced by EGF. In MIA PaCa-2 cancer cell line, somatostatin reverses the stimulatory effect of EGF on the phosphorylation of the tyrosine kinase portion of the EGF receptor (Hierowski et al. 1985). Some of our superactive analogs of somatostatin such as RC-160 and RC-121 exhibit even higher activity on dephosphorylation of the EGF receptor in MIA PaCa-2 line. Somatostatin analogs might inhibit pancreatic cancers by suppressing the action or secretion of gastrointestinal hormones and endogenous growth factors.

Inhibition of the growth of pancreatic acinar and ductal carcinomas in animal models by analogs of hypothalamic hormones was first reported by Redding and Schally (1984). The agonist [D-Trp^6]-LH-RH given daily or injected once a month in the form of controlled-release microcapsules, significantly decreased tumor weight and volume and suppressed serum testosterone levels. Chronic administration of some early somatostatin analogs also inhibited the growth of acinar pancreatic carcinomas in rats and of ductal cancers in hamsters (Gonzalez-Barcera et al. 1986, 1989; Redding and Schally 1984; Schally et al. 1984; Szende et al. 1990). Modern somatostatin analogs such as RC-121 and RC-160 (D-Phe-Cys-Tyr-D-Trp-Lys-Val-Cys-Trp-NH$_2$) also inhibited the growth of transplanted or BOP-induced ductal pancreatic cancers in male or female hamsters (Paz-Bouza et al. 1987). Recently, Zalatnai and Schally (1989) reported inhibition of tumor growth and evidence of histological regression of the BOP-induced pancreatic cancer in male hamsters after treatment with microcapsules of [D-Trp^6]-LH-RH or the somatostatin analog RC-160. The combination of both peptides produced the best results in terms of prolongation of survival and histological regressive changes.

Conclusion

It is apparent from our data, and findings of others, that several mechanisms may be involved in the controlling the growth of pancreatic cancers. Administration of somatostatin analogs slows the growth of the pancreatic tumor, possibly by inhibiting the secretion and/or action of gastrointestinal hormones and growth factors. LH-RH agonists decrease pancreatic tumor growth by eliminating the stimulatory effect of sex steroids. Combined administration of a modern somatostatin analog and an LH-RH agonist using long-acting delivery systems might induce a greater inhibition of cancer of the pancreas than the LH-RH agonist alone. Long-acting delivery systems for [D-Trp^6]-LH-RH based on microcapsules injectable once a month have been developed and used successfully (Zalatnai and Schally 1988). Similar systems for somatostatin analogs have been perfected recently. This combination of [D-Trp^6]-LH-RH microcapsules and a somatostatin analog will be the object of clinical trials in patients with pancreatic cancer; LH-RH antagonists could be also tried. A similar approach could also be tried in colorectal cancer, since sex steroids, gastrointestinal hormones, and growth factors may be involved in the tumorigenesis of the colon.

Use of the traditional methods of oncological surgery, i.e., resecting local disease and the pathways of its local spread and nodal metastases, provides only ineffective treatment of pancreatic cancer because the disease is usually systemic by the time of diagnosis. Although the new approach to the treatment with agonistic or antagonistic analogs of LH-RH alone or in combination with the new octapeptide analogs of somatostatin such as RC-160 is still in its early stages of development, it might prolong survival and improve quality of life for this dismal and virtually untreatable malignancy.

References

Anonymous (1986) Early diagnosis and screening for pancreatic cancer (editorial). Lancet ii:785–786

Bauer W, Briner W, Doepfner W, Haller R, Huguenin R, Marbach P, Petcher TJ, Pless J (1982) SMS-201-995: a very potent and selective octapeptide analogue of somatostatin with prolongued action. Life Sci 31:1133–1140

Benz C, Hollander C, Miller B (1986) Endocrine-responsive pancreatic carcinoma: steroid binding and cytotoxicity studies in human tumor cell lines. Cancer Res 46:2276

Blind PJ, Dahlgren ST (1987) Serum levels of the carbohydrate antigen CA-50 in pancreatic disease. Acta Chir Scand 153:45–49

Cai RZ, Szoke B, Lu R, Fu D, Redding TW, Schally AV (1986) Synthesis and biological activity of highly potent octapeptide analogs of somatostatin. Proc Natl Acad Sci USA 83:1896–1900

Cai RZ, Karashima T, Guoth J, Szoke B, Olsen D, Schally AV (1987) Superactive octapeptide somatostatin analogs containing tryptophan residue in position 1. Proc Natl Acad Sci USA 84:2502–2506

Chester JF, Gaissert HA, Ross JS, Malt RA (1986) Pancreatic cancer in the Syrian hamster induced by N-Nitrobis(2-oxopropyl)amine: cocarcinogenic effect of epidermal growth factor. Cancer Res 46:2954–2957

Comaru-Schally AM, Schally AV (1988) LH-RH agonists as adjuncts to somatostatin analogs in the treatment of pancreatic cancer. In: Lunenfeld B, Vickery B (eds) International symposium on Gn-RH analogues in cancer and human reproduction. MTP Press, Geneva

Connolly MM, Dawson PJ, Michelassi F, Moossa AR, Lowenstein F (1987) Survival in 1001 patients with carcinoma of the pancreas. Ann Surg 206:386

Corbishley TP, Iqbal MJ, Wilkinson ML, Williams R (1986) Androgen receptor in human normal and malignant pancreatic tissue and cell lines. Cancer 57:1992

Dembinski AB, Johnson LR (1980) Stimulation of pancreatic growth by secretin cerulein and pentagastrin. Endocrinology 106:323–328

Douglass HO Jr (1987) Pancreatic cancer: nihilism is obsolete! Pancreas 2:230–232

Fekete M, Zalatnai A, Comaru-Schally AM (1989) Membrane receptors for peptides in experimental and human pancreatic cancers. Pancreas 4:521–528

Gonzalez-Barcena D, Rangel-Garcia NE, Perez-Sanchez PL, Gutierrez-Samperio C, Garcia-Carrasco F, Comaru-Schally AM, Schally AV (1986) Response to D-Trp[6]-LH-RH in advanced adenocarcinoma of pancreas. Lancet ii:154

Gonzalez-Barcena D, Ibarra-Olmos MA, Garcia-Carrasco F, Gutierrez-Samperio C, Comaru-Schally AM, Schally AV (1989) Influence of D-Trp[6]-LH-RH on the survival time in patients with advanced pancreatic cancer. Biomed Pharmacother 43:1–5

Goustin AS, Leof EB, Shipley GD, Moses HL (1986) Growth factors and cancer. Cancer Res 46:1015–1029

Greenberger JJ, Toskes PP, Isselbacher KJ (1987) Diseases of the pancreas. In: Braunwald E, Isselbacher KJ, Petersdorf RG, Wilson JD, Martin JB, Fauci AS (eds) Harrison's principles of internal medicine, 11th edn. MacGraw-Hill, New York, pp 1372–1383

Greenway B, Duke D, Pym B, Iqbal MJ, Johnson PJ, Williams R (1982) The control of human pancreatic adenocarcinoma xenografts in nude mice by hormone therapy. Br J Surg 69:595

Hierowski MT, Liebow C, Du Spain K, Schally AV (1985) Stimulation by somatostatin of dephosphorylation of membrane proteins in pancreatic cancer MIA PaCa-2 cell line. FEBS Lett 179:252–256

Johnson LR (1981) Effects of gastrointestinal hormones on pancreatic growth. Cancer 47:1640–1645

Kalser MH, Ellenberg SS (Gastrointestinal Tumor Study Group) (1985) Pancreatic cancer: adjuvant combined radiation and chemotherapy following curative resection. Arch Surg 120:899

Konturek SJ, Tasler J, Obtulowicz W, Coy DH, Schally AV (1976) Effect of growth hormone releasing inhibiting hormone on hormones stimulating exocrine pancreatic secretion. J Clin Invest 58:1–6

Korc M, Magun BE (1985) Recycling of epidermal growth factor in a human pancreatic carcinoma cell line. Proc Natl Acad Sci USA 82:6172–6175

Malt RA (1983) Treatment of pancreatic cancer. JAMA 250:1433–1437

Moossa AR, Dawson PJ, Franklin WA, Udekwu AO, Lavella-Jones M (1986) Tumors of the pancreas. In: Moossa AR, Robson MC, Schimpff SC (eds) Comprehensive textbook of oncology. Williams and Wilkins, Baltimore, pp 1105–1132

Paz-Bouza JI, Redding TW, Schally AV (1987) Treatment of nitrosamine-induced pancreatic tumors in hamsters with analogs of somatostatin and luteinising hormone-releasing hormone. Proc Natl Acad Sci USA 84:1112–1116

Pollard MH, Anderson WAD, Brooks FP, Cohn I Jr, Copeland MM, Connelly RR, Fortner JG, Kissane JM, Lemon HM, Palmer PES, Thomas LB, Webster PD, Carter S (1981) Staging of cancer of pancreas. Cancer of the pancreas task force. Cancer 47:1631

Pousette A, Carlstrom K, Skoldefors H, Wilding N, Theve NO (1982) Purification of partial characterization of 178-estradiol binding macromolecules in the human pancreas. Cancer Res 42:633

Redding TW, Schally AV (1984) Inhibition of growth of pancreatic carcinoma in animal models by analogs of hypothalamic hormones. Proc Natl Acad Sci USA 81:248

Schally AV, Redding TW (1987) Somatostatin analogues as adjuncts to agonists of luteinizing hormone-releasing hormone in the treatment of experimental prostate cancer. Proc Natl Acad Sci USA 84:7275–7279

Schally AV, Comaru-Schally AM, Redding TW (1984) Antitumor effects of analogs of hypothalamic hormones in endocrine-dependent cancers. Proc Soc Ex Biol Med 175:259–281

Setyono-Han B, Henkelman MS, Foekens JA, Klijn JGM (1987) Direct inhibitory effects of somatostatin (analogues) on the growth of human breast cancer cells. Cancer Res 47:1566–1570

Skibber JM, Weiss SM, Mohiuddin M, Rosate FE (1985) Impact of radiotherapy on palliative gastroenterostomy in pancreatic cancer. Ann Surg 202:725

Szende B, Srkalovic G, Schally AV, Lapis K, Groot K (1990) Inhibitory effects of analogs of luteinizing hormone-releasing hormone and somatostatin on pancreatic cancers in hamsters. Cancer 65:2279–2290

Theve NO, Pousette A, Carlström K (1983) Adenocarcinoma of the pancreas – a hormone-sensitive tumor? A preliminary report on novaldex treatment. Clin Oncol 9:193–197

Zalatnai A, Schally AV (1989) Responsiveness of the hamster pancreatic cancer to treatment with microcapsules of D-Trp[6]-LH-RH and somatostatin analog RC-160: histological evidence of improvement. Int J Pancreatol 4:149–160

LH-RH Antagonists

LH-RH Antagonists:
State of the Art and Future Perspectives

G. F. Weinbauer and E. Nieschlag

Institut für Reproduktionsmedizin der Universität, WHO Kollaborationszentrum
zur Erforschung der männlichen Fertilität, Steinfurterstraße 107, W-4400 Münster, FRG

Introduction

Luteinizing hormone-releasing hormone (LH-RH) is produced in hypothalamic nuclei, travels via the portal blood to the anterior pituitary, and acts on gonadotropic cells by inducing the synthesis and release of luteinizing hormone (LH) and follicle-stimulating hormone (FSH). The gonadotropic hormones, in turn, regulate gonadal steroid production and gametogenesis. Reproductive functions, therefore, are critically dependent on LH-RH whose stimulatory effects are determined by its pulsatile release pattern (Knobil 1980) and by the availability of high-affinity binding sites at the pituitary site (Clayton and Catt 1981). Consequently, interference with the binding of native LH-RH to its pituitary receptors will provoke alterations of gonadal functions.

About 20 years ago, the amino acid sequence of the decapeptide LH-RH was revealed (Burgus et al. 1972; Matsuo et al. 1971), ultimately disclosing the relevance of each of the ten amino acids for the biological function of the LH-RH molecule. The most important amino acids are those in positions 1–3, which account for the hormone-releasing activity, and in positions 6 and 10, which determine receptor binding (Schally and Coy 1983; Sandow and König 1979). In addition, the peptide bonds between amino acids in positions 5–6 and 9–10 represent important sites for endopeptidase cleavage and degradation of the LH-RH molecule (Carone et al. 1987). Modifications of amino acids in relevant positions resulted in potent LH-RH analogs with agonistic or antagonistic actions relative to the native hormone.

By now probably more than 3000 LH-RH analogs have been synthesized. Whereas the LH-RH agonists have already found clinical application in the therapy of gonadal steroid-associated disease (Conn and Crowley 1991, for review), the LH-RH antagonists have not yet reached this stage. In this chapter, we review the development, mechanism of antigonadotropic and antigonadal action, current status and future issues of LH-RH antagonists.

Recent Results in Cancer Research, Vol. 124
© Springer-Verlag Berlin · Heidelberg 1992

Design of LH-RH Antagonists

Enormous efforts by several research groups were needed to develop active LH-RH antagonists, since suitable amino acid substituents and amino acid combinations had to be identified by empirical testing. This topic has been the subject of an extensive review by Karten and Rivier (1986). The observation that the potency of LH-RH antagonists, when assessed by their ability to block ovulation in the rat model, generally increased with increasing numbers of amino acid substitutions was a pivotal step towards synthesis of potent LH-RH antagonists. Furthermore, the use of hydrophobic D-amino acids greatly improved the activity of LH-RH antagonists, probably through enhancing stability and resistance to enzymatic degradation of the LH-RH analogs (Flouret et al. 1984). Substitution by basic D-amino acids in position 6 largely increased the antiovulatory activity (Coy et al. 1982).

Earlier LH-RH antagonists had four amino acid substitutions (4F-LH-RH antagonist, Nal-Arg-LH-RH antagonist), whereas "modern" antagonists of LH-RH are characterized by 5–7 amino acid modifications compared to the native hormone (Fig. 1). The compounds presented in Fig. 1 have already undergone clinical testing or are scheduled for clinical trials, namely 4F-LH-RH antagonist (Rivier and Vale 1981), Nal-Arg-LH-RH antagonist (Rivier et al. 1984), detirelix (Nestor et al. 1984), Nal-Glu-LH-RH antagonist (Rivier et al. 1986), antide (Nal-Lys; Ljungqvist et al. 1987), RS 26306 (Nestor et al. 1988), hoe 013 (Sandow et al. 1990a), and cetrorelix (SB-75, Bajusz et al. 1988a). The majority of LH-RH antagonists are characterized by D amino acids in positions 1–3 (avoiding the native LH-RH biological effect), and in positions 6 and 10 (related to LH-RH receptor binding and peptide degradation). Common to recent compounds are the amino acids acetyl-D-naphthylalanine in position 1, D-chlorophenylalanine in position 2, D-pyridylalanine or D-tryptophane in position 3 and D-alanine in position 10, except for the hoe 013 compound which has azaglycine in position 10.

Modification of amino acid in position 6 became an important issue when it became evident that LH-RH antagonists with D-arginine in this position induced local skin reactions at the sites of injection, i.e., the compounds Nal-Arg (Rivier et al. 1984) and detirelix (Nestor et al. 1984). Current amino acid substituents in position 6 are D-glutamine(anisole adduct) (Nal-Glu-LH-RH antagonist), D-nicotinoyllysine (antide), D-citrulline (cetrorelix) or D-serine (rhamnose) (hoe 013). For the compound RS 26306 a D-homoarginine was introduced in position 8 to shield the positive charge of arginine (quoted from Karten et al. 1990), leading to a substantial reduction in the histamine-releasing property of the substance (Lee et al. 1989). Conformationally constrained LH-RH antagonists were reported to be highly active in antiovulatory assays (Struthers et al. 1990). The potential of this class of LH-RH antagonists for suppression of pituitary-gonadal function has to be clarified in future studies.

With respect to the amino acid substitutions, the LH-RH antagonists are markedly different from the agonists (Fig. 1). These LH-RH analogs possess

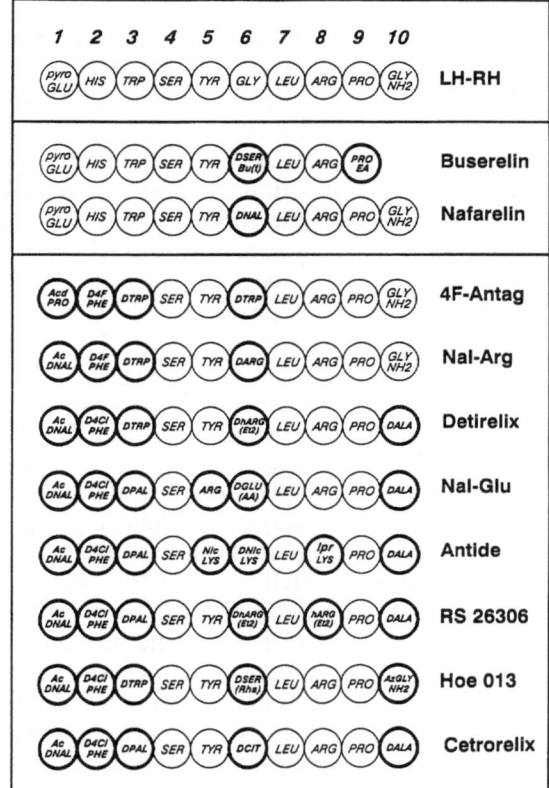

Fig. 1. Amino acid sequences of native LH-RH, two LH-RH agonists (buserelin and nafarelin) and eight LH-RH antagonists

either just one modification in position 6 or an additional change in position 10. The LH-RH agonists buserelin and nafarelin are given as representative examples.

Antigonadotropic Activity of LH-RH Antagonists

Mechanism of Action

Antagonists of LH-RH show a much higher affinity to the hypophyseal LH-RH binding sites than native LH-RH (Clayton and Catt 1980) and compete with endogenous LH-RH at the LH-RH receptor. Blockade of the pituitary LH-RH receptors, leading to prevention of the stimulatory effects of LH-RH, is the mechanism underlying the antigonadotropic and antigonadal effects of LH-RH antagonists (Heber et al. 1982; Rivier et al. 1980).

Most of the available evidence would suggest that LH-RH antagonists prevent LH-RH action at the pituitary level by competitive LH-RH receptor occupancy rather than by a down-regulation of LH-RH binding sites. This view is supported by the observations that even after prolonged exposure of gonadotropic cells to radiolabeled LH-RH antagonists, most of the label remained outside the cells (Loumaye et al. 1984; Morel et al. 1987; Wynn et al. 1986), that an LH-RH antagonist did not affect de novo synthesis of LH-RH receptors in vitro (Braden and Conn 1990), and that the in vitro LH-RH-induced LH/FSH stimulation could be dose-dependently blocked by an LH-RH antagonist and vice versa (Franchimont et al. 1991). Deleterious effects of an LH-RH antagonist on gonadotropic cells as a possible cause of the antigonadotropic effect have recently been ruled out (Danforth et al. 1991a).

Following chronic exposure to LH-RH antagonists, pituitary binding of labeled agonists was reduced to 5% – 10% of control (Rea et al. 1986; Puente and Catt 1986). This loss of binding capacity of the pituitary most likely represents LH-RH receptor occupancy rather than true loss, since it has been demonstrated that dissociation of the LH-RH antagonist from its receptor restored LH-RH binding (Clayton et al. 1982). In this context, the LH-RH antagonists appear quite different from agonists, which are known to induce internalization of the receptor-ligand complex (Duello et al. 1983) and LH-RH receptor down-regulation (Loumaye and Catt 1983; McNeilly et al. 1991). According to Skralovich et al. (1990), pituitary LH-RH receptor up- and down-regulation were induced by the compound cetrorelix released from a depot preparation. The issue of whether LH-RH antagonists do in fact alter hypophyseal LH-RH receptor numbers still remains to be resolved.

The view that LH-RH antagonists are indeed competitors of LH-RH rather than down-regulatory substances also receives substantial support from in vivo studies on the ability of exogenously administered synthetic LH-RH to restore LH-RH antagonist-induced inhibition of LH secretion. Following acute administration of LH-RH antagonist to male monkeys, pituitary stimulation tests using different LH-RH doses at different time intervals after LH-RH antagonist injection elicited a LH-RH dose-dependent LH release in relation to the duration of LH inhibition (Marshall et al. 1986a). In female monkeys, the LH response to a given dose of LH-RH decreased with increasing doses of LH-RH antagonist (Chillik et al. 1987; Leal et al. 1989a). The ability of LH-RH to overcome LH-RH antagonist-induced inhibition of LH release, compatible with the view of a competitive blockade of LH-RH binding sites, was also documented in recent clinical studies (Hall et al. 1990; Lahlou et al. 1990).

The suppressive effect of LH-RH antagonists on anterior pituitary hormone secretion is most pronounced for LH and FSH. However, an inhibitory effect of LH-RH antagonists on prolactin secretion has been observed in female monkeys (Geisthövel et al. 1988; Olive et al. 1989) and in clinical studies (Urban et al. 1988). Inhibitory effects of LH-RH antagonists on prolactin levels were not observed in cultured pituitary from male rats (Franchimont et al. 1991), in male cynomolgus monkeys (G. F. Weinbauer and E. Nieschlag, unpublished observations) and in normal men (Pavlou et al. 1990a). These authors, however, reported a significant increase of growth hormone releasing hormone (GH-RH)-stimulated growth hormone (GH) release during LH-RH antagonist administration.

Preclinical and Clinical Evaluation

In nonhuman primate models, the antagonists of LH-RH provoked a precipitous decline of LH and gonadal steroid hormone secretion within several hours (Adams et al. 1986; Akhtar et al. 1985; Kenigsberg et al. 1984; Leal et al. 1988; Weinbauer et al. 1984, 1988, 1989) and were devoid of the initial burst of hormone secretion typical for the LH-RH agonists.

In the early 1980s the first clinical studies reported inhibitory effects of LH-RH antagonists on LH and FSH secretion in women (Zarate et al. 1981) and in men (Gonzalez-Barcena et al. 1980). Subsequent studies using the compounds Nal-Arg, detirelix, or the 4F-LH-RH antagonist further substantiated the antigonadotropic potential of LH-RH antagonists in a clinical setting (Cetel et al. 1983; Dahl et al. 1986; Hall et al. 1988, 1990; Pavlou et al. 1986, 1987a, b). Davis et al. (1987) demonstrated inhibitory effects of the compound [Ac-D-4-Cl-Phe^{1,2}, D-Trp^3, D-Lys^6, D-Ala^{10}]-LH-RH in postmenopausal women. These compounds, however, were either not sufficiently active in eliminating gonadotropic hormone secretion and/or caused irritations at the sites of injection forcing discontinuation from more extensive clinical evaluation.

The majority of clinical investigations with LH-RH antagonists employed the Nal-Glu compound. Suppression of LH and, although to a lesser extent, of FSH release was achieved with 15–150 µg/kg of Nal-Glu in normal women (Hall et al. 1990) and with 10–300 µg/kg in postmenopausal women (Mortola et al. 1989; Urban et al. 1988). The duration of the antigonadotropic action of Nal-Glu increased with the dose administered. Inhibition of LH secretion in normal men for 24 h and longer required a single dose of at least 5 mg/volunteer (Jockenhövel et al. 1988; Pavlou et al. 1989; Salameh et al. 1991; Tenover et al. 1990). Daily administration of 5 mg for 21 days (Salameh et al. 1991) or 75 µg/kg for 10 days (Bagatell et al. 1989) evoked sustained supression of LH and FSH release. Initial rebounds encountered within the first few days of LH-RH antagonist administration could be overcome by 12-hourly administration of 5 mg Nal-Glu (Pavlou et al. 1989).

Improvement of the antigonadotropic potency was achieved with the compounds antide (Ljungqvist et al. 1987) and cetrorelix (Bajusz et al. 1988a). Preclinical studies in monkeys (Leal et al. 1988; Weinbauer and Nieschlag 1990a) comparing the antigonadotropic activity of Nal-Glu and antide, revealed that antide was considerably longer-acting than Nal-Glu. In addition, cetrorelix appeared even longer-acting than antide (Weinbauer and Nieschlag 1990a). To date, data from clinical evaluations are available for cetrorelix and RS 26306.

Phase I clinical trials with cetrorelix were conducted by Brensing et al. (1991) and Behre et al. (1991). In the latter investigation normal male volunteers received a single subcutaneous injection of cetrorelix over a dose range of 0.25–5.0 mg. At doses of 1 mg and higher, cetrorelix significantly lowered serum concentrations of LH and testosterone in a cetrorelix-dose-dependent manner. At the highest dose of 5 mg testosterone secretion remained suppressed for 24–36 h. Maximal suppression of LH and testosterone levels at the 2 and 5 mg doses occurred after 6 and 12 h, respectively. Release of immunoactive FSH was not significantly altered. Injections of cetrorelix were well tolerated, and transient local erythema, unrelated to the dose of LH-RH antagonist, was encountered only occasionally. No local induration or pruritus nor any adverse systemic side effect was noted in any volunteer. This LH-RH antagonist was similarly potent to the Nal-Glu compound but was clearly superior in terms of side effects. Recently another LH-RH antagonist, RS 26306, given as a single subcutaneous injection, was reported to inhibit gonadotropin and testosterone secretion with minimal erythema seen at the injection site (Gaitan et al. 1991).

LH-RH Antagonists Versus LH-RH Agonists

Although both classes of LH-RH analogs bind to the same hypophyseal LH-RH receptor, they induce quite divergent effects on the secretion, expression, and molecular composition of gonadotropic hormones and their subunits. As already mentioned, LH-RH antagonists merely block the LH-RH receptor, which is followed by a precipitous decline in gonadotropin release, whereas LH-RH agonists transiently stimulate gonadotropin secretion, which is followed by down-regulation of LH-RH receptors. Suppression of secretion of bioactive and immunoactive LH is achieved with both LH-RH agonists (Akhtar et al. 1983; Bhasin et al. 1987; Meldrum et al. 1984) and LH-RH antagonists (Weinbauer and Nieschlag 1985; Khurshid et al. 1991; Pavlou et al. 1990 b; Lindner et al. 1990).

Remarkable differences between LH-RH antagonists and agonists, however, were observed with regard to the bio- and immunoactivity of the FSH molecule. The antagonistic analogs markedly lowered serum levels of immunoactive FSH (Couzinet et al. 1991; Khurshid et al. 1991; Salameh et al. 1991) and bioactive FSH (Dahl et al. 1986; Kessel et al. 1988), with FSH bioactivity being even more affected than immunoactivity (Dahl et al. 1988). The relative insensitivity of immunoactive FSH in some clinical trials is possibly related to nonparallelisms between immuno- and bioassay (Jockenhövel et al. 1990). With GnRH agonists the suppression of immunoactive FSH release was incomplete or transient (Behre et al. 1992; Huhtaniemi et al. 1984; Santen et al. 1984) and, more importantly, FSH bioactivity remained nearly unaffected (Huhtaniemi et al. 1988; Pavlou et al. 1988). Similarly, in patients suffering from pituitary tumors, LH-RH antagonist treatment reduced FSH and α-subunit secretion (Danesdhoost et al. 1990), whereas with LH-RH agonists LH/FSH and α-subunit levels remained unaltered (Daneshdoost et al. 1990) or were even stimulated (Klibanski et al. 1989; Roman et al. 1984). The evaluation of LH-RH antagonists for their potential to reduce pituitary adenoma size has been suggested. The molecular mechanisms leading to the disparate effects of LH-RH analogs on pituitary gonadotropic hormones/subunits are not understood. These analogs, however, are valuable tools for studying LH-RH-dependent regulation of gonadotropin subunit assembly in vitro and in vivo.

Antigonadal Activity of LH-RH Antagonists

Basic Studies

In sufficient doses LH-RH antagonists very effectively interrupted oogenesis, spermatogenesis, and fertility in laboratory animal models. Administration of LH-RH antagonists to male rats (Arslan et al. 1989; Bhasin et al. 1988; Rivier et al. 1981) or to female rats (Nekola and Coy 1984; Bokser et al. 1991) induced gonadal involution and infertility which was completely reversible after cessation of LH-RH treatment. The histological appearance of the testes (decreased tubular diameter, loss of spermatids) and the ovaries (predominance of small follicles, absence of corpora lutea) is typical of the consequences of withdrawal of trophic hormones. No evidence of detrimental effects of LH-RH antagonists at the gonadal level has been found.

In adult male cynomolgus monkeys (*Macaca fascicularis*) we evaluated in detail the effects of different LH-RH antagonists (ORG 30276, detirelix, Nal-Glu and antide) on the size and spermatogenic function of the testes (Akhtar et al. 1985; Weinbauer et al. 1984, 1988, 1991 a, b). Daily doses of LH-RH antagonists between 350 and 460 µg/kg were administered for periods of 9–16 weeks. Testicular size was reduced by 4 weeks and reached nadir values of 15% – 25% of baseline within 8–16 weeks (Fig. 2). Azoospermia was achieved within 7–12 weeks of LH-RH antagonist administration. The success rate of azoospermia was 85%, underscoring the suitability of LH-RH antagonists for suppression of pituitary-gonadal function in primates.

At the testicular level, first alterations of germ cell organization were already seen after 4 weeks of LH-RH antagonist treatment (Weinbauer et al. 1991 a), including the beginning of disorganisation of the germinal epithelium and the appearance of degenerating germ cells. By 8 weeks a marked germ cell loss was encountered which encompassed mainly the more advanced germ cells (Fig. 2). Between 9 and 16 weeks of LH-RH antagonist treatment, varying degrees of germinal epithelium involution were present. In maximally involuted seminiferous tubules, spermatogonia were the predominating germinal cells (Fig. 3). Accumulation of lipids and lysosomal activity in Sertoli cell cytoplasm indicated phagocytosis of degenerating germ cells similar to that observed previously with LH-RH agonists (Weinbauer et al. 1987 b). Qualitatively, the histological picture of the testes was comparable to that seen after hypophysectomy or LH-RH agonist administration (Marshall et al. 1986 b; Weinbauer et al. 1987 a). In spite of the long-lasting hypogonadotropic state,

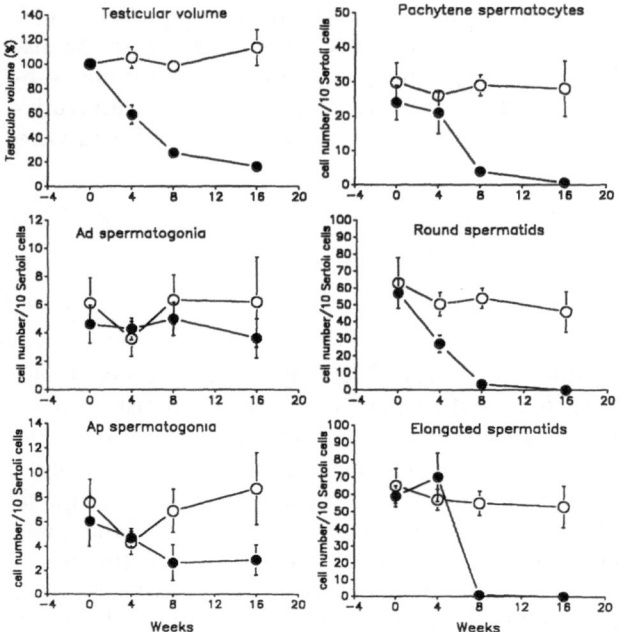

Fig. 2. Quantitative effects of long-term LH-RH antagonist treatment on testicular size and germ cell population in adult monkeys. Groups of five animals received vehicle (*open circles*) or 450 µg/kg per day of antide (*filled symbols*). Note that the numbers of A-dark (*Ad*) spermatogonia, which represent pool of reserve stem cells for germ cell proliferation, remained unaltered (*Ap*, A-pale). Data modified from Weinbauer et al. (1991a)

only the number of the A-pale spermatogonia (the renewing testicular germ cells) was reduced, whereas the A-dark spermatogonia (the testicular reserve stem cells) remained unaffected. The persistence of the testicular reserve stem cells even after prolonged LH-RH antagonist-induced gonadotropin deficiency provides the basis for recovery of the germinal epithelium. Destructive alterations in testicular architecture were not encountered.

Testicular dimensions and sperm counts fully recovered after cessation of LH-RH antagonist administration, indicating that the LH-RH antagonist-induced inhibitory effects on primate gonads are completely reversible (Fig. 4). Direct antigonadal actions of LH-RH analogs are extremely unlikely because of the absence of binding sites for LH-RH in primate gonads (Asch et al. 1981; Clayton and Huhtaniemi 1982). This is supported by the findings that in vitro incubation of Leydig cells from monkey testes with LH-RH antagonist (Mann et al. 1989) or from human testes with LH-RH agonists (Rajfer et al. 1987; Namiki et al. 1987) did not affect human chorionic gonadotropin (hCG) induced testosterone production.

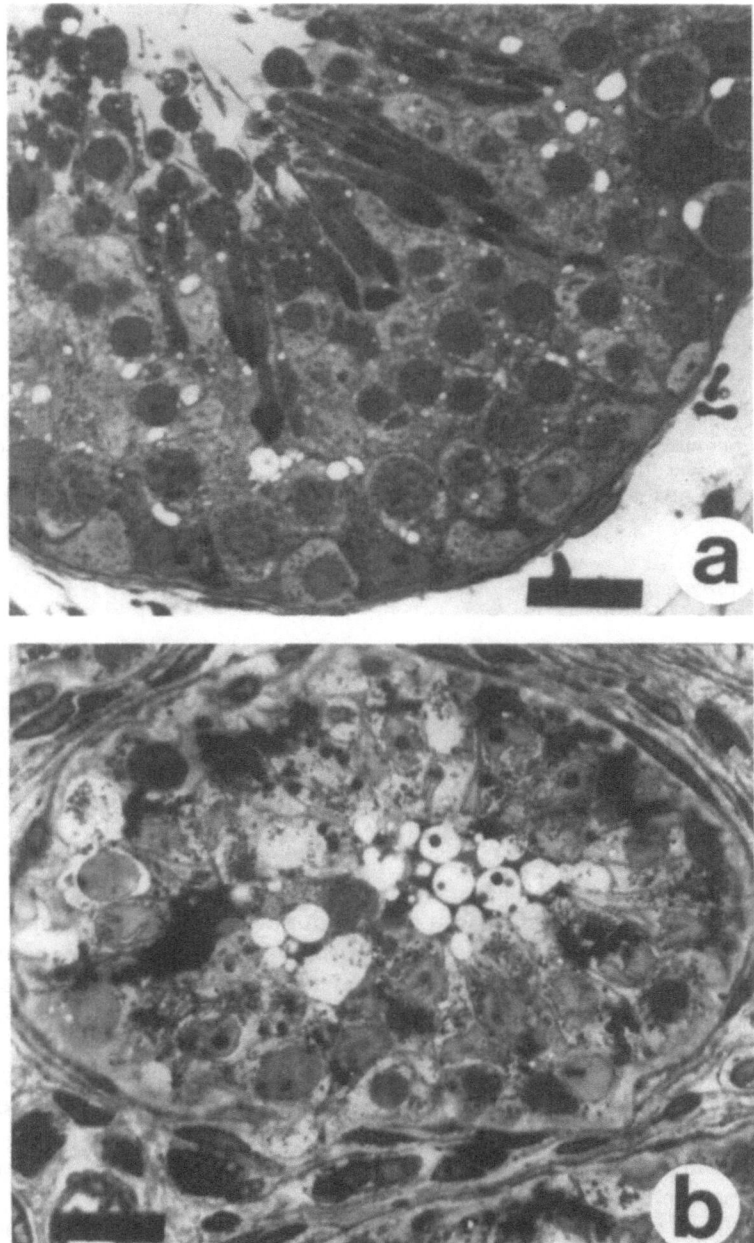

Fig. 3 a, b. Morphology of the seminiferous epithelium following 16 weeks of treatment with (a) vehicle or (b) 450 µg/kg per day of antide in adult monkeys. Normal and complete spermatogenesis is present in vehicle-treated testes. Seminiferous tubule diameter is markedly reduced. The predominating germ cells are spermatogonia. Leydig cells (*bottom left on* b) contain lipid droplets. No destructive alterations are present. *Bar,* 15 µm

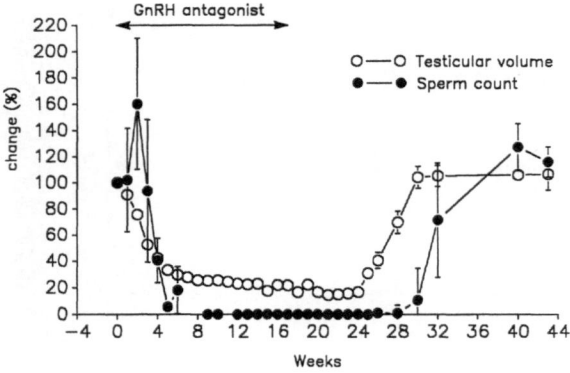

Fig. 4. Percentage changes of testicular size and sperm counts of five adult monkeys receiving high-dose LH-RH antagonist treatment (900 µg/kg per day of antide) for 18 weeks. The pronounced and long-lasting inhibitory effects of the LH-RH antagonist were completely reversible after cessation of treatment

Contraceptive Studies

The pronounced and reversible suppression of gonadal function in nonhuman primate models by the LH-RH antagonists raised hopes that these compounds might open a new avenue towards the development of an endocrine contraceptive. In the male, induction of a hypogonadotropic state by LH-RH antagonists for the purpose of suppressing spermatogenesis necessitates the simultaneous provision of androgens to avoid the large spectrum of androgen-deficiency symptoms (Nieschlag et al. 1989). In a first preclinical study in monkeys, testosterone was provided via Silastic capsules concomitantly with LH-RH antagonist treatment (Weinbauer et al. 1987c). Although severe oligozoospermia could be induced in three out of four animals, comparison with a previous study (Weinbauer et al. 1984) suggested a slight attenuating effect of androgen supplementation on LH-RH antagonist-induced spermatogenic involution. Subsequently, a more comprehensive study was performed (Weinbauer et al. 1988) which comprised two doses of a long-acting testosterone ester (Weinbauer et al. 1986). Evaluation of sperm counts and testicular histology clearly demonstrated that in a dose-dependent manner testosterone prevented the induction of azoospermia by the LH-RH antagonist (Nal-Glu). Although animals in the testosterone-substituted groups were extremely oligozoospermic, consistent azoospermia could not be induced.

Since observations in the rat indicated that the ability of androgens to maintain testicular function is greater than for reinitiation of the process (Harris et al. 1977), the effects of LH-RH antagonist and delayed androgen substitution were evaluated in the nonhuman primate model (Weinbauer et al. 1989). Testosterone administration (corresponding to the lower dose of the previous study) was given from the sixth week of LH-RH antagonist treatment, thus comprising approximately one length of the spermatogenic cycle of macaque monkeys (Clermont 1972). The total study duration was 18 weeks. In spite of androgen supplementation, azoospermia was achieved by week 9 in nine monkeys and during week 13 in the tenth animal; azoospermia persisted throughout the entire LH-RH antagonist administration phase and for another 7–13 weeks thereafter. In contrast to our studies, a recent publication reported achievement of azoospermia by concomitant LH-RH antagonist and testosterone treatment (Bremner et al. 1991). Testosterone substitution was provided via testosterone-filled Silastic capsules which maintained serum testosterone concentrations at baseline levels. In our previous study (Weinbauer et al. 1988) concentrations of serum testosterone were in the upper normal range and were provided from an ester preparation. Moreover, in the study by Bremner et al. (1991), sperm counts of monkeys were rather low and increased during the experimental period. The animals used in our studies were fully adult. Whether this difference in animals and design can account for the differences observed remains a subject of speculation.

This model of LH-RH antagonist and delayed testosterone administration, as developed in the monkey (Weinbauer et al. 1989), has been used in two clinical trials for male contraception (Table 1). In study 1, eight normal men received the LH-RH antagonist Nal-Glu for 16 weeks at a daily dose of 7.5 mg. Androgen substitution was delayed by 2 weeks and consisted of 150 mg testosterone enanthate given every 2 weeks (Tom et al. 1991). In seven out of the eight subjects, azoospermia was achieved within 6–8 weeks of LH-RH antagonist administration. One volunteer developed welts at the sites of injection and discontinued the trial in week 12. Baseline sperm counts were attained 10–12 weeks after withdrawal of the LH-RH antagonist. In study 2, 8 normal men were subjected to 10 mg Nal-Glu/day for 20 weeks (Pavlou 1991). Testosterone enanthate was given at 25 mg/week starting 2 weeks later than Nal-Glu treatment. Sperm counts began to decline in week 4 and azoospermia was induced in seven subjects within 6–12 weeks. The remaining volunteer was severely oligozoospermic. These first clinical evaluations render LH-RH

Table 1. Male contraceptive trials with a LH-RH antagonist

	Study 1[a]	Study 2[b]
LH-RH antagonist	Nal-Glu	Nal-Glu
Mode of administration	subcutaneous	subcutaneous
Dose (mg/day)	7.5	10.0
Subjects (*n*)	8	8
Duration of treatment (weeks)	16	20
Androgen substitution (TE, start in week 3)	150 mg/2 weeks	25 mg/week
Rate of azoospermia	7/8	7/8
Recovery of semen parameters (%)	100	100

TE, testosterone enanthate (intramuscular injection).
[a] Study 1; Tom et al. (1991).
[b] Study 2, Pavlou (1991).

antagonists, unlike the GnRH agonists (Behre et al. 1992; Weinbauer et al. 1990), as highly promising agents for male fertility regulation.

The ability of LH-RH antagonists to block ovulation and corpus luteum function was also demonstrated in monkeys (Fraser et al. 1985, 1987; Gordon et al. 1991; Kenigsberg and Hodgen 1986) and recently in women with normal menstrual cycles (Marshall et al. 1991). The LH-RH antagonist detirelix was given at a dose of 5 mg every other day for a period of 27 days. This treatment regimen interrupted follicular development and blocked ovulation as judged by serum progesterone levels. After termination of treatment a LH surge occurred within 10–16 days. Due to low estrogen levels hot flushes were experienced by some women.

Pharmacokinetics and Pharmacodynamics of LH-RH Antagonists

Single or multiple injections of potent LH-RH antagonists resulted in long-lasting inhibitory effects on the pituitary-gonadal axis. The duration of the suppressive action of LH-RH antagonists was clearly dose-dependent and is an important parameter for distinguishing the potency of LH-RH antagonists. Animal studies with LH-RH antagonists revealed an extremely long duration of antigonadotropic action. Following daily treatment with 3 mg/kg antide for 6 days to ovariectomized monkeys, it took 100 (!) days for LH and FSH secretion to recover to baseline (Leal et al. 1989 b). Administration of 3 mg/kg antide, given as a single injection, maintained bioactive antide levels – assessed in rat pituitary cultures – for more than 30 days (Danforth et al. 1991 b). A single dose of 6 mg/kg antide in male rats suppressed testosterone for at least 5 weeks (Habenicht et al. 1990) and a dose of 2 mg/kg administered to rats on days 0 (proestrus), 3, 6, and 9 abolished fertility for 156 days (Sharpe et al. 1990). Clinical trials with antide have not been conducted so far.

The compound cetrorelix, which is already clinically available, also proved to be very long-acting in the orchiectomized nonhuman primate model (Weinbauer and Nieschlag 1990 a). After a single subcutaneous dose of 5 mg, the terminal half-life of cetrorelix was 29.1 ± 3.9 h (Behre et al. 1991) compared with 12.8 ± 2.7 h for the same dose of Nal-Glu (Pavlou et al. 1989). The prolonged duration of action of LH-RH antagonists has been attributed to their binding to circulating proteins (Davis et al. 1987; Danforth et al. 1990). This might explain why the plasma half-lives of LH-RH antagonists were found to increase with higher doses of LH-RH antagonists in monkeys (Chan et al. 1988) and in women (Davis et al. 1987). It must be recalled here, however, that LH-RH and LH-RH agonists also bind to plasma proteins although to a different extent (20%–30% for LH-RH versus 70%–80% for nafarelin; Chan and Chaplin 1985). In addition, the hydrophobicity of LH-RH antagonists might facilitate the formation of depots at the sites of injection.

Although the clinically relevant LH-RH antagonists exhibited a favorable pharmacokinetic profile, an effective and sustained suppression of hormone levels in males required daily injection of 5 mg or more of the substance. Depot preparations loaded with LH-RH antagonists analogous to those already available for LH-RH agonists are the method of choice to improve the pharmacodynamic properties of LH-RH antagonists. Such development is mandatory to make the clinical use of LH-RH antagonists feasible and attractive, and first experimental studies demonstrated the activity of LH-RH antagonist-loaded depot formulations. Polylactic-glycolide depot preparations (single injection) released biologically active cetrorelix for 20–40 days in rats (Bokser et al. 1990; Csernus et al. 1990). A constant release preparation of hoe 013 was active for 2 weeks (Sandow et al. 1990b). Continuous release of an LH-RH antagonist appeared more effective in suppressing testicular weights than daily injection (50 µg/day via an osmotic minipump versus 2×25 µg/day) in nude mice (Redding and Schally 1990; Szende et al. 1990a). It has been estimated that a constant release preparation requires only about a tenth of the amount of injected substance to achieve a comparable effect (Sandow et al. 1990b).

Side Effects of LH-RH Antagonists

Chronic administration of LH-RH antagonists for 9–18 weeks to male monkeys resulted in body weight reduction amounting to 4%–20% of baseline in individual animals (Bremner et al. 1991; Weinbauer and Nieschlag 1990b). These effects of LH-RH antagonist treatment are most likely related to androgen deficiency and could be prevented by androgen substitution. Food and water intake remained unaffected (Weinbauer et al. 1987c).

Rodent studies revealed that some the LH-RH antagonists caused anaphylactoid reactions (Phillips et al. 1988), hypotension (Limonta et al. 1985), skin lesions following intradermal injection (Hahn et al. 1985), and formation of edema (Schmidt et al. 1984). Histamine-induced release from mast cells by the LH-RH antagonists was at least partially responsible for the observed side effects and related to the presence of D-arginine in position 6 (Morgan et al. 1986). Side effects such as local irritation due to histamine release at the size of injection were also encountered in clinical trials with LH-RH antagonists (Nal-Arg, detirelix, Nal-Glu). The development of safer LH-RH antagonists focused on increasing their antigonadotropic potency and minimizing their histamin-releasing properties (Karten et al. 1990).

Widespread clinical application of the LH-RH antagonist Nal-Glu is prohibited by the local side-effects associated with it such as induration or pruritus. Markedly reduced edematogenic and anaphylactoid effects compared with Nal-Glu were described for the LH-RH antagonists antide (Phillips et al. 1988; Ljungqvist et al. 1987), cetrorelix (Bajusz et al. 1988b), RS 26306 (Lee et al. 1989) and hoe 013 (Sandow et al. 1990a). In clinical studies cetrorelix administration induced only a transient local erythema at the injection site that was not dose-related, did not emerge consistently, and disappeared within 30 min (Behre et al. 1991; Brensing et al. 1991). Minimal local side effects were also reported in recent clinical trials with the compound RS 26306 (Gaitan et al. 1991) and with hoe 013 in experimental animals (Sandow et al. 1990b).

Untoward systemic side effects were not encountered in any clinical study. The occurrence of local side effects is probably inherent to LH-RH antagonist (analog) injection, but appeared rather moderate with improved compounds. Conceivably, spreading the daily dose over 24 h by means of depot preparations might considerably reduce the incidence of local side effects.

Future Perspectives of LH-RH Antagonists

Therapy of Gonadal Steroid-Associated Disease

Therapeutic studies with LH-RH antagonists have not been undertaken up to now. Basically, LH-RH antagonists should be appropriate for the therapy of any disease that can be treated with a LH-RH agonist, i.e., precocious puberty, endometriosis, polycystic ovarian syndrome, uterine fibroids, breast and ovarian cancer, and prostatic cancer. GnRH antagonists might be useful in conditions when the initial stimulation of gonadal steroid secretion, imposed by the LH-RH agonists, is clinically undesirable. Aggravation of disease symptoms ("flare-up") during the initial phase of LH-RH agonist therapy has been noted in some patients with advanced stage of prostatic cancer (Parmar et al. 1985; Waxman 1989). Initial combination therapy with cyproterone acetate (Boccon-Gibod et al. 1986; de Voogt et al. 1990) or flutamide (Lunglmayr 1989; Waxman 1989) has been used to avoid the flare-up. High doses of a LH-RH antagonist were able to blunt and even prevent the GnRH agonist-induced hypersecretion of bioactive LH and testosterone in a nonhuman primate model (Sharma et al. 1992). This might represent another approach to avoid the LH-RH agonist-associated flare-up in certain patients.

Animal studies demonstrated the ability of LH-RH antagonists to inhibit the growth of a variety of experimentally induced tumors, i.e., prostatic tumor (Habenicht et al. 1990; Szepeshazi et al. 1991), mammary tumors (Szende et al. 1990 a; Reissmann et al. 1992; Sandow et al. 1990 b) and pancreatic tumors (Szende et al. 1990 b). According to Szepeshazi et al. (1991), who compared depot formulations of LH-RH antagonist and agonist, the reduction of prostatic tumor (Dunning) weight required approximately the threefold amount of LH-RH antagonist compared with agonist. Growth inhibition of a pancreatic tumor was achieved by constant release of either LH-RH agonist or antagonist at equal doses (8 µg/day for 60 days; Szende et al. 1990 b). On the other hand, comparing cetrorelix and D-Trp[6] at a daily dose of 25 µg/day and both administered as a depot formulation, cetrorelix was more potent than the LH-RH agonist or ovariectomy in decreasing growth of a mouse mammary tumor (Szende et al. 1990 a).

The rationale for the clinical use of LH-RH antagonists would be based on the assumption that the lack of the initial stimulation of gonadal steroid hormone release might result in a better and/or earlier responses compared with LH-RH agonists. Potential benefits of initial blockade of androgen action during LH-RH agonist therapy of prostatic cancer have been extensively studied. Conflicting results (Crawford and Allen 1990; de Voogt et al. 1990; Robinson et al. 1990) might be partially explained by a differential hormonal dependence of tumor tissue in early and advanced disease states. Nonetheless, LH-RH antagonists would permit a straightforward possibility of evaluating the effects of immediate and complete withdrawal of gonadal steroids on tumor development. Based on their precipitous inhibitory action, the LH-RH antagonists might prove useful for shortening the treatment length in women with benign gynecological disease, i.e., endometriosis and myoma uteri.

Potential for Contraception

Besides long-acting testosterone esters (WHO 1990), at present LH-RH antagonists are the most promising candidates for male fertility control. Their acceptability will be crucial to the mode of administration, i.e., long-lasting and biodegradable release preparations. Appropriately long-acting testosterone esters are already available at least for experimental use (Weinbauer et al. 1986). Agonistic analogs of LH-RH suppressed testicular function only in the absence of androgen substitution (Frick and Aulitzky 1986). In the presence of testosterone, which is necessary to avoid androgen-deficiency, LH-RH agonists failed to induce consistent azoospermia and cannot be considered for male contraception (Behre et al. 1992; Weinbauer et al. 1990). Aside from possible stimulatory effects of androgens on testicular function (Weinbauer and Nieschlag 1990 c), the inability of LH-RH agonists to suppress the bioactivity of FSH might also be important, since FSH is a key regulator of primate spermatogenesis (Matsumoto 1989; Marshall and Nieschlag 1987; Weinbauer et al. 1991 a, b).

For female contraception, the use of LH-RH analogs will require estrogen supplementation to prevent hot flushes and, more importantly, osteoporosis. The combination of LH-RH analogs and estrogen and progesterone is reminiscent of the female contraceptive pill already available. A recent report, however, claims that GnRH agonists plus estrogen and intermittent progesterone would markedly reduce the risk of life-time breast cancer occurrence (Spicer et al. 1991). The prospects for LH-RH antagonists as female contraceptives appear rather limited in view of the already available choices. To prevent the LH surge in ovarian hyperstimulation protocols, however, the immediate inhibitory effects of LH-RH antagonists on LH/estradiol levels might prove useful.

Concluding Remarks

Antagonists of LH-RH can suppress gonadotropin release in humans and act, almost certainly, through competitive occupancy of the pituitary LH-RH receptor. Gonadal function can be reversibly inhibited, and LH-RH antagonists proved highly promising as potential male contraceptive agents. The possibility that LH-RH antagonists will be superior to LH-RH agonist therapy of gonadal steroid-associated disease awaits clinical proof. Unlike "earlier" LH-RH antagonists, "modern" compounds are quite safe and induce only minimal, local side effects at the injection sites. At present, LH-RH antagonists are administered by daily subcutaneous injections in clinical trials. Sustained release formulations for LH-RH antagonists are urgently required to make clinical use feasible. Such preparations might, in addition, help to reduce the currently high doses of LH-RH antagonist required for continued suppression of pituitary and gonadal function and may induce fewer local side effects.

References

Adams LA, Bremner WJ, Nestor JJ Jr, Vickery BH, Steiner RA (1986) Suppression of plasma gonadotropins and testosterone in adult male monkeys (Macaca fascicularis) by a potent inhibitory analog of gonadotropin-releasing hormone. J Clin Endocrinol Metab 62:58–63

Akhtar FB, Marshall GR, Wickings EJ, Nieschlag E (1983) Reversible induction of azoospermia in rhesus monkeys by constant infusion of a GnRH agonist using osmotic minipumps. J Clin Endocrinol Metab 56:534–540

Akhtar FB, Weinbauer GF, Nieschlag E (1985) Acute and chronic effects of a gonadotrophin-releasing hormone antagonist on pituitary function in monkeys. J Endocrinol 104:345–354

Arslan M, Weinbauer GF, Khan SA, Nieschlag E (1989) Testosterone and dihydrotestosterone, but not estradiol, selectively maintain pituitary and serum follicle-stimulating hormone in gonadotropin-releasing hormone antagonist treated male rats. Neuroendocrinology 49:395–401

Asch RH, van Sickle M, Rettori V, Balmaceda JP, Eddy CA, Coy DH, Schally AV (1981) Absence of LH-RH binding sites in corpora lutea from rhesus monkeys (Macaca mulatta). J Clin Endocrinol Metab 53:215–217

Bagatell CJ, McLachlan RI, de Kretser DM, Burger HG, Vale WW, Rivier J, Bremner WJ (1989) A comparison of the suppressive effects of testosterone and a potent new gonadotropin-releasing hormone antagonist on gonadotropin and inhibin levels in normal men. J Clin Endocrinol Metab 69:43–48

Bajusz S, Scernus VJ, Janaky T, Bokser L, Fekete M, Schally AV (1988a) New antagonists of LH-RH: II. Inhibition and potentiation of LH-RH by closely related analogues. Int J Pept Protein Res 32:425–435

Bajusz S, Kovacs M, Gazdag M, Bokser L, Karashima T, Csernus VJ, Janaky T, Guoth J, Schally AV (1988b) Highly potent antagonists of luteinizing hormone-releasing hormone free of edematogenic effects. Proc Natl Acad Sci USA 85:1637–1641

Behre HM, Klein B, Steinmeyer E, Nieschlag E (1991) Effective suppression of luteinizing hormone and testosterone by single doses of the new gonadotropin-releasing hormone antagonist SB-75 in normal men. 73rd annual meeting of the Endocrine Society, Washington, June 12–15 (abstract 1155)

Behre HM, Nashan D, Hubert W, Nieschlag E (1992) Depot GnRH agonist blunts the androgen-induced suppression of spermatogenesis in a clinical trial for male contraception. J Clin Endocrinol Metab 74:84–90

Bhasin S, Yuan QX, Steiner BS, Swerdloff RS (1987) Hormonal effects of gonadotropin-releasing hormone (GnRH) agonist in men: effects of long term treatment with GnRH agonist infusion and androgen. J Clin Endocrinol Metab 65:568–574

Bhasin S, Fielder T, Peacock N, SodMoriah UA, Swerdloff RS (1988) Dissociating antifertility effects of GnRH antagonists from its adverse effects on mating behavior in male rats. Am J Physiol 32:E84–E91

Boccon-Gibod L, Laudat MH, Dugue MA, Steg A (1986) Cyproterone acetate prevents initial rise of serum testosterone induced by luteinizing hormone-releasing hormone analogs in the treatment of metastatic carcinoma of the prostate. Eur Urol 12:400–402

Bokser L, Bajusz S, Groot K, Schally AV (1990) Prolonged inhibition of luteinizing hormone and testosterone levels in male rats with the luteinizing hormone-releasing hormone antagonist SB-75. Proc Natl Acad Sci USA 87:7100–7104

Bokser L, Skralovic G, Szepeshazi K, Schally AV (1991) Recovery of pituitary-gonadal function in male and female rats after prolonged administration of a potent antagonist of luteinizing hormone-releasing hormone (SB-75). Neuroendocrinology 54:136–145

Braden TD, Conn PM (1990) Altered rate of synthesis of gonadotropin-releasing hormone receptors: effects of homologous hormone appear independent of extracellular calcium. Endocrinology 126:2577–2582

Bremner WJ, Bagatell CJ, Steiner RA (1991) Gonadotropin-releasing hormone antagonist plus testosterone: a potential male contraceptive. J Clin Endocrinol Metab 73:465–469

Brensing KA, Schepke M, Enzweiler CH, Lademacher CH, Klingmüller D (1991) The new GnRH antagonist ("SB-75") induced a safe and effective testosterone suppression in normal men: a phase I study. Acta Endocrinol (Copenh) 124:9 (abstr)

Burgus R, Butcher M, Amoss M, Ling N, Monahan MW, Rivier J, Fellows T, Blackwell R, Vale W, Guillemin R (1972) Primary structure of the ovine hypothalamic luteinizing hormone-releasing hormone factor (LRF). Proc Natl Acad Sci USA 69:278–285

Carone FA, Stetler-Stevenson MA, May V, LaBarbera A, Flouret G (1987) Differences between in vitro and in vivo degradation of LH-RH by rat brain and other organs. Am J Physiol 253:E317–E321

Cetel NS, Rivier J, Vale W, Yen SSC (1983) The dynamics of gonadotropin inhibition in women induced by an antagonistic analog of gonadotropin-releasing hormone. J Clin Endocrinol Metab 57:62–65

Chan RL, Chaplin MD (1985) Plasma binding of LH-RH and nafarelin acetate, a highly potent LH-RH agonist. Biochem Biophys Res Commun 127:673–679

Chan RL, Ho W, Webb AS, LaFargue JA, Nerenberg CA (1988) Disposition of Detirelix, a potent luteinizing hormone-releasing hormone antagonist, in rat and monkeys. Pharm Res 5:335–340

Chillik CF, Itskovitz J, Hahn DW, McGuire JL, Danforth DR, Hodgen GD (1987) Characterizing pituitary response to a gonadotropin-releasing hormone (GnRH) antagonist in monkeys: tonic follicle-stimulating hormone/luteinizing hormone secretion versus acute GnRH challenge tests before, during and after treatment. Fertil Steril 48:480–485

Clayton RN, Catt KJ (1980) Receptor-binding affinity of gonadotropin-releasing hormone analogs: analysis by radioligand-receptor assay. Endocrinology 106:1154–1159

Clayton RN, Catt KJ (1981) Gonadotropin-releasing hormone receptors: characterization, physiological regulation and relationship to reproductive function. Endocr Rev 2:186–209

Clayton R, Huhtaniemi I (1982) Absence of gonadotropin-releasing hormone receptors in human gonadal tissue. Nature 299:56–59

Clayton RN, Channabasavaiah K, Stewart JM, Catt KJ (1982) Hypothalamic regulation of pituitary gonadotropin-releasing hormone receptors: effects of hypothalamic lesions and a gonadotropin-releasing hormone antagonist. Endocrinology 110:1108–1115

Clermont Y (1972) Kinetics of spermatogenesis in mammals: seminiferous epithelium cycle and spermatogonial renewal. Physiol Rev 52:198–236

Conn PM, Crowley WF Jr (1991) Gonadotropin-releasing hormone and its analogues. N Engl J Med 324:93–103

Couzinet B, Lahlou N, Thomas G, Thalabard JC, Bouchard P, Roger M, Schaison G (1991) Effects of gonadotrophin releasing hormone antagonist and agonist on the pulsatile release of gonadotrophins and alpha-subunit in postmenopausal women. Clin Endocrinol (Oxf) 34:477–483

Coy DH, Horvath A, Nekola MV, Coy EJ, Erchegyi J, Schally AV (1982) Peptide antagonists of LH-RH: large increases in antiovulatory activities produced by basic D-amino acids in the six position. Endocrinology 110:1445–1449

Crawford ED, Allen JA (1990) Treatment of newly diagnosed state D2 prostate cancer with leuprolide and flutamide or leuprolide alone, phase III, Intergroup study 0036. J Steroid Biochem Mol Biol 37:961–963

Csernus VJ, Szende B, Groot K, Redding TW, Schally AV (1990) Development of a radioimmunoassay for a potent luteinizing hormone-releasing hormone antagonist. Drug Res 40:111–118

Dahl KD, Pavlou SN, Kovacs WJ, Hsueh AJW (1986) The changing ratio of serum bioactive to immunoreactive follicle-stimulating hormone in normal men following treatment with gonadotropin releasing hormone antagonist. J Clin Endocrinol Metab 63:792–794

Dahl KD, Bicsak TA, Hsueh AJW (1988) Naturally occurring antihormones: secretion of FSH antagonists by women treated with a GnRH analog. Science 239:72–74

Daneshdoost L, Pavlou SN, Molitch ME, Gennarelli TA, Savino PJ, Sergott RC, Bosley TM, Rivier JE, Vale WV, Snyder PJ (1990) Inhibition of follicle-stimulating hormone secretion from gonadotroph adenomas by repetitive administration of a gonadotropin-releasing hormone antagonist. J Clin Endocrinol Metab 71:92–97

Danforth DR, Gordon K, Leal JA, Williams RF, Hodgen GD (1990) Extended presence of antide (Nal-Lys GnRH antagonist) in circulation: prolonged duration of gonadotropin inhibition may derive from antide binding to serum proteins. J Clin Endocrinol Metab 70:554–556

Danforth DR, Williams RF, Gordon K, Hodgen GD (1991a) Inhibition of pituitary gonadotropin secretion by the gonadotropin-releasing hormone antagonist antide: I. In vitro studies on mechanism of action. Endocrinology 128:2036–2040

Danforth DR, Williams RF, Gordon K, Leal JA, Hodgen GD (1991b) Inhibition of pituitary gonadotropin secretion by the gonadotropin-releasing hormone antagonist antide: II. Development of an in vitro bioassay for characterization of pharmacokinetics and pharmacodynamics of antide in circulation. Endocrinology 128:2041–2044

Davis MR, Veldhuis JD, Rogol AD, Dufau ML, Catt KJ (1987) Sustained inhibitory actions of a potent antagonist of gonadotropin-releasing hormone in postmenopausal women. J Clin Endocrinol Metab 64:1268–1274

de Voogt HJ, Klijn JGM, Studer U, Schröder F, Sylvester R, de Pauw M (1990) Orchidectomy versus buserelin in combination with cyproterone acetate, for 2 weeks or continuously, in the treatment of metastatic prostatic cancer. Preliminary results of EORTC-trial 30843. J Steroid Biochem Mol Biol 37:965–969

Duello TM, Nett TM, Farquhar MG (1983) Fate of a gonadotropin-releasing hormone agonist internalized by rat pituitary gonadotrophs. Endocrinology 112:1–10

Flouret G, Stettler-Stevenson MA, Carone FA, Peterson DR (1984) Enzymatic degradation of LH-RH and analogs. In: Vickery BH, Nestor JJ Jr, Hafez ESE (eds) LH-RH and its analogs. MTP Press, Lancaster, pp 397–410

Franchimont P, Almer SM, Charlet-Renard CJ, Daubresse CL, Kicovic PP (1991) Effects of a novel gonadotropin-releasing hormone antagonist (ORG 30850) on gonadotropin and prolactin secretion by rat pituitary cells in culture. Acta Endocrinol (Copenh) 124:98–106

Fraser HM, Baird DT, McRae GI, Nestor JJ Jr, Vickery BH (1985) Suppression of luteal progesterone secretion in the stumptailed macaque by an antagonist analogue of luteinizing hormone-releasing hormone. J Endocrinol 104:R1–R4

Fraser HM, Nestor JJ Jr, Vickery BH (1987) Suppression of the luteal function by a luteinizing hormone-releasing hormone antagonist during the early luteal phase in the stumptailed macaque monkey and the effects of subsequent administration of human chorionic gonadotropin. Endocrinology 121:612–618

Frick J, Aulitzky W (1986) Effects of a potent LH-RH agonist on the pituitary gonadal axis with and without testosterone substitution. Urol Res 14:261–264

Gaitan D, Lindner J, Farley MG, Monroe SE, Pavlou SN (1991) Antireproductive properties of a novel GnRH antagonist in men. 73rd annual meeting of the Endocrine Society, Washington, June 12–15 (Abstract 1156)

Geisthövel F, Arana JB, Balmaceda JP, Tojas FJ, Asch RH (1988) Prolactin and gonadotrophin dynamics in response to antagonists of LH-RH and dopamine in ovarectomized rhesus monkeys: a dissection of their common secretion. Hum Reprod 3:591–595

Gonzalez-Barcena D, Ortiz HT, Gordon F, Kastin AJ, Coy D, Schally AV (1980) Influence of LH-RH agonists and antagonists on gonadotropin release in humans. Int J Fertil 25:185–189

Gordon K, Williams RF, Danforth DR, Hodgen GD (1991) Antide-induced suppression of pituitary gonadotropin and ovarian steroid secretion in cynomolgus monkeys. Premature luteolysis and prolonged inhibition of folliculogenesis following single treatment. Biol Reprod 44:701–706

Habenicht UF, Schneider MR, El Etreby MF (1990) Effect of the new potent LH-RH antagonist antide. J Steroid Biochem Mol Biol 37:937–942

Hahn DW, McGuire JL, Vale WV, Rivier J (1985) Reproductive/endocrine and anaphylactoid properties of an LH-RH-antagonist, ORF 18260 [Ac-DNal[1](2), 4FDPhe[2], D-Trp[3], D-Arg[6]]-GnRH. Life Sci 37:505–514

Hall JE, Brodie TD, Badger TM, Rivier JE, Vale WV, Conn PM, Schoenfeld, Crowley WF Jr (1988) Evidence of differential control of FSH and LH secretion by gonadotropin-releasing hormone (GnRH) from the use of a GnRH antagonist. J Clin Endocrinol Metab 67:524–531

Hall JE, Whitcomb RW, Rivier JE, Vale WV, Crowley WF Jr (1990) Differential regulation of luteinizing hormone, follicle-stimulating hormone, and free alpha-subunit secretion from the gonadotrope by gonadotropin-releasing hormone (GnRH): evidence from the use of two GnRH antagonists. J Clin Endocrinol Metab 70:328–335

Harris ME, Bartke A, Weisz J, Watson D (1977) Effects of testosterone and dihydrotestosterone on spermatogenesis, rete testis fluid, and peripheral androgen levels in hypophysectomized rats. Fertil Steril 28:1113–1117

Heber D, Dodson R, Swerdloff RS, Channabasavaiah K, Stewart JM (1982) Pituitary receptor site blockade by a gonadotropin-releasing hormone antagonist in vivo: mechanism of action. Science 216:420–421

Huhtaniemi IT, Stewart JM, Channabasavaiah K, Fraser HM, Clayton RN (1984) Effect of treatment with GnRH antagonist, GnRH antiserum and bromocriptine on pituitary-testicular function of adult rats. Mol Cell Endocrinol 34:127–135

Huhtaniemi IT, Dahl KD, Rannikko S, Hsueh AJ (1988) Serum bioactive and immunoreactive follicle-stimulating hormone in prostatic cancer patients during gonadotropin-releasing hormone agonist treatment and after orchidectomy. J Clin Endocrinol Metab 66:308–313

Jockenhövel F, Bhasin S, Steiner B, Rivier JE, Vale WV, Swerdloff RS (1988) Hormonal effects of single gonadotropin-releasing hormone antagonist doses in men. J Clin Endocrinol Metab 66:1065–1070

Jockenhövel F, Khan SA, Niechlag E (1990) Varying dose-response characteristics of different immunoassays and an in vitro bioassay for FSH are responsible for changing ratios of biologically active to immunologically active FSH. J Endocrinol 127:523–532

Karten MJ, Rivier J (1986) Gonadotrophin-releasing hormone analog design. Structure-function towards the development of agonists and antagonists: rationale and perspective. Endocr Rev 7:44–66

Karten MJ, Hoeger CA, Hook WA, Lindberg MC, Naqvi RH (1990) The development of safer GnRH antagonists: strategy and status. In: Bouchard P, Haour F, Franchimont P, Schatz B (eds) Recent progress on GnRH and gonadal peptides. Elsevier, Paris, pp 147–158

Kenigsberg D, Hodgen GD (1986) Ovulation inhibition by administration of weekly gonadotropin-releasing hormone antagonist. J Clin Endocrinol Metab 62:734–738

Kenigsberg D, Littman BA, Hodgen GD (1984) Medical hypophysectomy: I. Dose-response using a gonadotropin-releasing hormone antagonist. Fertil Steril 42:112–115

Kessel B, Dahl KD, Kazer RR, Liu CH, Rivier J, Vale W, Hsueh AJW, Yen SSC (1988) The dependency of bioactive follicle-stimulating hormone secretion on gonadotropin-releasing hormone in hypogonadal and cycling women. J Clin Endocrinol Metab 66:361–366

Khurshid S, Weinbauer GF, Nieschlag E (1991) Effects of testosterone and gonadotropin-releasing hormone (GnRH) antagonist on basal and GnRH-stimulated gonadotrophin-secretion in orchidectomized monkeys. J Endocrinol 129:363–370

Klibanski A, Jameson JL, Killer BMK, Crowley WF Jr, Zervas NT, Rivier J, Vale WV, Bikkal H (1989) Gonadotropin and alpha-subunit responses to chronic gonadotropin-releasing hormone analog administration in patients with glycoprotein hormone-secreting tumors. J Clin Endocrinol Metab 68:81–86

Knobil E (1980) The neuroendocrine control of the menstrual cycle. Recent Prog Horm Res 36:53–88

Lahlou N, Delivet S, Bardin CW, Roger M, Spitz IM, Bouchard P (1990) Changes in gonadotropin and alpha-subunit after a single administration of gonadotropin-releasing hormone antagonist in adult males. Fertil Steril 53:898–905

Leal JA, Williams RF, Danforth DR, Gordon K, Hodgen GD (1988) Prolonged duration of gonadotropin inhibition by a third generation GnRH antagonist. J Clin Endocrinol Metab 67:1325–1327

Leal JA, Gordon K, Williams RF, Danforth DR, Roh SI, Hodgen GD (1989a) Probing studies on multiple dose effects of antide (Nal-Lys) GnRH antagonist in ovariectomized monkeys. Contraception 40:623–633

Leal JA, Williams RF, Danforth DR, Gordon K, Hodgen GD (1989b) Prolonged duration of gonadotropin inhibition by a third generation GnRH antagonist. J Clin Endocrinol Metab 67:1325–1327

Lee CH, Van Antwerp D, Hedley L, Nestor JJ Jr, Vickery BH (1989) Comparative studies on the hypotensive effect of LH-RH antagonists in anesthetized rats. Life Sci 45:697–702

Limonta P, Bardin CW, Ladishenskaya A, Pavlou S, Sundaram K, Thau RB (1985) Species differences in the sensitivity to a GnRH antagonist. Contraception 32:75–85

Lindner J, Rivier JE, Vale WV, Pavlou SN (1990) Regulation of pituitary glycoprotein alpha-subunit secretion after administration of a luteinizing hormone-releasing hormone antagonist in normal men. J Clin Endocrinol Metab 70:1216–1224

Ljungqvist A, Feng DM, Tang PFL, Kubota M, Okamoto Y, Zhang Y, Bowers CY, Hool WA, Folkers K (1987) Design, synthesis and bioassays of antagonists of LH-RH which have high antiovulatory activity and release negligible histamine. Biochem Biophys Res Comm 148:849–856

Loumaye E, Catt KJ (1983) Agonist-induced regulation of pituitary receptors for gonadotropin-releasing hormone. J Biol Chem 258:12002–12009

Loumaye E, Wynn PC, Coy D, Catt KJ (1984) Receptor-binding properties of gonadotropin-releasing hormone derivatives. J Biol Chem 259:12663–12671

Lunglmayr G (1989) "Zoladex" versus "Zoladex" plus flutamide in the treatment of advanced prostate cancer: first interim analysis of an international trial. In: Murphy GP, Khoury S (eds) Therapeutic progress in urological cancers. Liss, New York, pp 145–152 (Progress in clinical and biological research, Vol 303)

Mann DR, Adams SR, Gould KG, Orr TE, Collins DC (1989) Evaluation of the possible direct effects of gonadotrophin-releasing hormone analogues on the monkey (Macaca mulatta) testis. J Reprod Fertil 85:89–95

Marshall GR, Nieschlag E (1987) The role of FSH in male reproduction. In: Sheth AR (ed) Inhibins: isolation, estimation and physiology, vol 1. CRC Press, Boca Raton, Florida, pp 3–15

Marshall GR, Akhtar FB, Weinbauer GF, Nieschlag E (1986a) Gonadotrophin-releasing hormone (GnRH) overcomes GnRH antagonist-induced suppression of LH secretion in primates. J Endocrinol 110:145–150

Marshall GR, Jockenhövel F, Lüdecke D, Nieschlag E (1986b) Maintenance of complete but quantitatively reduced spermatogenesis in hypophysectomized monkeys by testosterone alone. Acta Endocrinol (Copenh) 113:424–431

Marshall LA, Fluker MR, Jaffe RB, Monroe SE (1991) Inhibition of follicular development by a potent antagonistic analog of gonadotropin-releasing hormone (detirelix). J Clin Endocrinol Metab 72:927–933

Matsumoto AM (1989) Hormonal control of spermatogenesis. In: Burger H, de Kretser DM (eds) The testis, 2nd edn. Raven, New York, pp 181–196

Matsuo H, Baba Y, Nair RM, Arimura A, Schally AV (1971) Structure of the porcine LH- and FSH-releasing hormone: I. The proposed amino acid sequence. Biochem Biophys Res Comm 43:1334–1339

McNeilly JR, Brown P, Clark AJ, McNeilly AS (1991) Gonadotrophin-releasing hormone modulation of gonadotrophins in the ewe: evidence for differential effects on gene expression and hormone secretion. J Mol Endocrinol 7:35–43

Meldrum DR, Tsao Z, Monroe SE, Braunstein GD, Sladek J, Lu JKH, Vale W, Rivier J, Judd HL, Chang RJ (1984) Stimulation of LH fragments with reduced bioactivity following GnRH agonist administration in women. J Clin Endocrinol Metab 58:755–757

Morel G, Dihl F, Aubert ML, Dubois PM (1987) Binding and internalization of native gonadoliberin (GnRH) by anterior pituitary gonadotrophs of the rat. A quantitative autoradiographic study after cryo-ultramicrotomy. Cell Tissue Res 248:541–550

Morgan JE, O'Neil CE, Coy DH, Hocart SJ, Nekola MV (1986) Antagonistic analogs of luteinizing hormone-releasing hormone are mast cell secretagogues. Int Arch Allergy Appl Immunol 80:70–75

Mortola JF, Sathanandam M, Pavlou SN, Dahl KD, Hsueh AJW, Rivier JE, Vale WV, Yen SSC (1989) Suppression of bioactive and immunoreactive follicle-stimulating hormone and luteinizing hormone levels by a potent gonadotropin-releasing hormone antagonist: pharmacodynamic studies. Fertil Steril 51:957–963

Namiki M, Sonoada T, Nonomura N, Nishimune Y, Nakamura M, Matsumoto K, Okuyama (1987) Effects of a gonadotropin-releasing hormone agonist analog (ICI 118630) on endocrine functions of human testis in vivo and in vitro. Fertil Steril 48:1012–1017

Nekola M, Coy DH (1984) LH-RH antagonists in females. In: Vickery BH, Nestor JJ Jr, Hafez ESE (eds) LH-RH and its analogs. MTP Press, Lancaster, pp 125–136

Nestor JJ Jr, Ho TL, Tahilramani R, McRae GI, Vickery BH (1984) Long-acting LH-RH agonists and antagonists. In: Vickery BH, Nestor JJ Jr, Hafez ESE (eds) LH-RH and its analogs. MTP Press, Lancester, pp 24–35

Nestor JJ Jr, Tahilramani R, Ho TL, Goodpasture JC, Vickery BH, Ferrandon P (1988) Design of luteinizing hormone-releasing hormone antagonists with reduced potential for side effects. In: Jung G (ed) Peptides 1988: proceedings of the 20th European Peptide Symposium. De Gruyter, Berlin, pp 592–594

Nieschlag E, Behre HM, Weinbauer GF (1989) Hormonal methods for the regulation of male fertility. In: Serio M (ed) Perspectives in andrology. Raven, New York, pp 517–529 (Serono symposia, vol 53)

Olive DL, Sabella V, Riehl RM, Schenken RS, Moreno A (1989) Gonadotropin-releasing hormone antagonists attenuate estrogen/progesterone-induced hyperprolactinemia in monkeys. Fertil Steril 51:1040–1045

Parmar H, Phillips RH, Lightman SL, Edwards L, Allen L, Schally AV (1985) Randomised controlled study of orchidectomy vs long-acting D-Trp[6]-LH-RH microcapsules in advanced prostatic carcinoma. Lancet ii:1201–1205

Pavlou SN (1991) GnRH antagonists in men: development of a male contraceptive. Tianjin international symposium on LH-RH analogues, Tianjng, China, September 24–26 (Abstract 33)

Pavlou SN, Devold CR, Island DP, Wakefield G, Rivier J, Vale W, Rabin D (1986) Single subcutaneous doses of a luteinizing hormone-releasing hormone antagonist suppress serum gonadotropin and testosterone levels in normal men. J Clin Endocrinol Metab 63:303–308

Pavlou SN, Interlandi JW, Wakefield G, Island DP, Rivier J, Vale W, Kovacs WJ (1987a) Gonadotropins and testosterone escape from suppression during prolonged luteinizing hormone-releasing hormone antagonist administration in normal men. J Clin Endocrinol Metab 64:1070–1074

Pavlou SN, Wakefield GB, Island DP, Hoffman PG, LePage ME, Chan RL, Nerenberg CA, Kovacs WJ (1987b) Suppression of pituitary-gonadal function by a potent new luteinizing hormone-releasing hormone antagonist in normal men. J Clin Endocrinol Metab 64:931–936

Pavlou SN, Dahl KD, Wakefield G, Rivier J, Vale W, Hsueh AJW, Lindner J (1988) Maintenance of the ratio of bioactive to immunoreactive follicle-stimulating hormone in normal men during chronic luteinizing-hormone agonist administration. J Clin Endocrinol Metab 66:1005–1009

Pavlou SN, Wakefield G, Schlechter NL, Lindner J, Souza KH, Kamilaris TC, Kondidaris S, Rivier JE, Vale WW, Toglia M (1989) Mode of suppression of pituitary and gonadal function after acute or prolonged administration of a luteinizing hormone-releasing hormone antagonist in normal men. J Clin Endocrinol Metab 68:446–454

Pavlou SN, DeBold CR, Orth DN (1990a) LH-RH antagonists: clinical studies in man. In: Bouchard P, Haour F, Franchimont P, Schatz B (eds) Recent progress on GnRH and gonadal peptides. Elsevier, Paris, pp 195–208

Pavlou SN, Veldhuis JD, Lindner J, Souza KH, Urban RJ, Rivier JE, Vale WW, Stallard DJ (1990b) Persistence of concordant luteinizing hormone (LH), testosterone, and alpha-subunit pulses after LH-releasing hormone antagonist administration in normal men. J Clin Endocrinol Metab 70:1472–1478

Phillips A, Hahn DW, McGuire JL, Ritchie D, Capetola RJ, Bowers C, Folkers K (1988) Evaluation of the anaphylactoid activity of a new LH-RH antagonist. Life Sci 43:883–888

Puente M, Catt KJ (1986) Inhibition of pituitary-gonadal function in male rats by a potent GnRH antagonist. J Steroid Biochem 25:917–925

Rajfer J, Sikka SC, Swerdloff RS (1987) Lack of a direct effect of gonadotropin hormone-releasing hormone agonist on human testicular steroidogenesis. J Clin Endocrinol Metab 64:62–67

Rea MA, Marshall GR, Weinbauer GF, Nieschlag E (1986) Testosterone maintains pituitary and serum FSH and spermatogenesis in gonadotrophin-releasing hormone antagonist-suppressed rats. J Endocrinol 108:101–107

Redding TW, Schally AV (1990) Inhibition of the pituitary-gonadal axis in nude male mice by continuous administration of LH-RH agonists and antagonists. J Endocrinol 126:309–315

Reissmann T, Hilgard P, Harleman JH, Engel J, Comaru-Schally AM, Schally AV (1992) Treatment of experimental DMBA induced mammary carcinoma with Cetrorelix (SB-75): a potent antagonist of luteinizing hormone-releasing hormone. J Cancer Res Clin Oncol 118:44–49

Rivier C, Vale W (1981) Temporal relationship between the abortifacient effects of GnRH antagonists and hormonal secretion. Biol Reprod 24:1061–1067

Rivier C, Rivier J, Vale W (1980) Antireproductive effects of a potent gonadotropin-releasing hormone antagonist in the male rat. Science 210:93–95

Rivier C, Rivier J, Vale W (1981) Effect of a potent GnRH antagonist and testosterone propionate on mating behaviour and fertility in the male rat. Endocrinology 108:1998–2001

Rivier JE, Rivier C, Perrin M, Porter J, Vale WW (1984) LH-RH analogs as antiovulatory agents. In: Vickery BH, Nestor JJ Jr, Hafez ESE (eds) LH-RH and its analogs. MTP Press, Lancaster, pp 11–22

Rivier JE, Porter J, Rivier CL, Perrin M, Corrigan A, Hook WA, Siraganian RP, Vale WW (1986) New effective gonadotropin-releasing hormone antagonists with minimal potency for histamine release in vitro. J Med Chem 29:1846–1851

Robinson DM, Mahler C, Smith PH, Keuppens F, De Moura JLC, Bono E, Newling D, Sylvester R, D Pauw R, Vermeylen K, Ongena P, members of the EORTC-GU Group (1990) Orchidectomy versus Zoladex plus Eulexin in patients with metastatic prostate cancer (EORTC 30853). J Steroid Biochem Mol Biol 37:951–959

Roman SH, Goldstein M, Kourides IA, Comite F, Bardin CW, Krieger DT (1984) The luteinizing hormone-releasing hormone (LH-RH) agonist D-Trp^6-Pro^9-NEt LH-RH increased rather than lowered LH and alpha-subunit levels in a patient with an LH-secreting tumor. J Clin Endocrinol Metab 58:313

Salameh W, Bhasin S, Steiner B, McAdams LA, Peterson M, Swerdloff RS (1991) Marked suppression of gonadotropins and testosterone by an antagonist analog of gonadotropin-releasing hormone in men. Fertil Steril 55:156–164

Sandow J, König W (1979) Studies with fragments of highly active analogue of luteinizing hormone releasing hormone. J Endocrinol 8:175–182

Sandow J, Stöckemann K, Jerabek-Sandow G (1990a) Pharmacokinetics and endocrine effects of slow release formulations of LH-RH analogues. J Steroid Biochem Mol Biol 37:925–931

Sandow J, Stöckemann K, Kibet PG, Lill NM, Neubauer H, Jerabek-Sandow G, Hahn M, Kille S (1990b) Effect of a new LH-RH antagonist on DMBA-induced mammary tumours. 2nd international symposium on "Hormonal manipulation of cancer: peptides, growth factors and new (anti)steroidal agents", Rotterdam, 9–11 April (Abstract 116). Eur J Cancer 26:175

Santen RJ, Demers LM, Max DT, Smith J, Stein BS, Glode LM (1984) Long term effects of administration of a gonadotropin-releasing hormone superagonist analog in men with prostatic carcinoma. J Clin Endocrinol Metab 58:397–400

Schally AV, Coy DH (1983) Stimulatory and inhibitory analogs of LH-releasing hormone. In: McCann SM, Dhindsa DS (eds) Role of peptides and proteins in control of reproduction. Elsevier, New York, pp 89–110

Schmidt F, Sundaram K, Thau RB, Bardin CW (1984) (Ac-D-Nal(2), 4FD-Phe2,D-Trp³,D-Arg⁶)-LH-RH, a potent antagonist of LH-RH, produces transient edema and behavioral changes in rats. Contraception 29:283–289

Sharma OP, Weinbauer GF, Behre HM, Nieschlag E (1992) The gonadotropin-releasing hormone (GnRH) agonist-induced initial rise of bioactive LH and testosterone secretion can be blocked in a dose-dependent manner by GnRH antagonist in the nonhuman primate. Urol Res (in press)

Sharpe KL, Bertero MC, Lyon BP, Muse KN, Vernon MW (1990) Follicular atresia and infertility in rats treated with gonadotropin-releasing hormone antagonist. Endocrinology 127:25–31

Srkalovic G, Bokser L, Radulovic S, Korkut E, Schally AV (1990) Receptors for luteinizing hormone-releasing hormone (LH-RH) in dunning R 3327 prostate cancers and rat anterior pituitaries after treatment with a sustained delivery system of LH-RH antagonist SB-75. Endocrinology 127:3052–3060

Spicer DV, Shoupe D, Pike MC (1991) GnRH agonists as contraceptive agents: predicted significantly reduced risk of breast cancer. Contraception 44:289–310

Struthers RS, Tanaka G, Koerber SC, Solmajer T, Baniak EL, Gierasch LM, Vale W, Rivier J, Halger AT (1990) Design of biologically active, conformationally constrained GnRH antagonists. Proteins 8:295–304

Szende B, Skralovic G, Groot K, Lapis K, Schally AV (1990a) Growth inhibition of mouse MIXT mammary tumor by the luteinizing hormone-releasing hormone antagonist SB-75. JNCI 82:513–517

Szende B, Srkalovic G, Groot K, Lapis K, Schally AV (1990b) Regression of nitrosamide-induced pancreatic cancers in hamsters treated with luteinizing hormone-releasing hormone antagonists or agonists. Cancer Res 50:3716–3721

Szepeshazi K, Korkut E, Szende B, Lapis K, Schally AV (1991) Histological changes in dunning prostate tumors and testes of rats treated with LH-RH antagonist SB-75. Prostate 18:255–270

Tenover JS, Dahl KD, Vale WV, Rivier JE (1990) Hormonal responses to a potent gonadotropin-releasing hormone antagonist in normal elderly men. J Clin Endocrinol Metab 71:881–888

Tom L, Salameh W, Bhasin S, Steiner B, Peterson M, Swerdloff RS (1991) Male contraception: achievement of reversible azoospermia by combined gonadotropin releasing hormone antagonist and testosterone treatment. 73rd annual meeting of the Endocrine Society, Washington, June 12–15 (Abstract 1154)

Urban RJ, Pavlou SN, Rivier JE, Vale W, Daufau ML, Veldhuis JD (1988) Suppressive actions of a gonadotropin-releasing hormone antagonist on luteinizing hormone, follicle-stimulating hormone, and prolactin release in estrogen-deficient postmenopausal women. Am J Obstet Gynecol 162:1255–1260

Waxman J (1989) Short-term anti-androgen therapy and very long-acting depot gonadotropin-releasing hormone agonist for prostatic cancer. In: Murphy GP, Khoury S (eds) Therapeutic progress in urological cancers. Liss, New York, pp 61–68 (Progress in clinical and biological research, vol 303)

Weinbauer GF, Nieschlag E (1985) Regulation of primate testicular function by GnRH analogues. Med Biol 63:210–217

Weinbauer GF, Nieschlag E (1990a) Evaluation of the antigonadotropic activity of different GnRH antagonists in the nonhuman primate. Gynecol Endocrinol 4:21 (abstr)

Weinbauer GF, Nieschlag E (1990b) The role of testosterone in spermatogenesis. In: Nieschlag E, Behre HM (eds) Testosterone. Action, deficiency, substitution. Springer, Berlin Heidelberg New York, pp 23–50

Weinbauer GF, Nieschlag E (1990c) Preclinical studies with GnRH antagonists. In: Maggi M, Geenen V (eds) Horizons in endocrinology. Raven, New York, pp 287–296

Weinbauer GF, Surmann FJ, Akhtar FB, Shah GV, Vickery BH, Nieschlag E (1984) Reversible inhibition of testicular function by a gonadotropin-releasing hormone antagonist in monkeys (Macaca fascicularis). Fertil Steril 42:906–914

Weinbauer GF, Marshall GR, Nieschlag E (1986) New injectable testosterone ester maintains serum testosterone of castrated monkeys in the normal range for four months. Acta Endocrinol (Copenh) 113:128–132

Weinbauer GF, Respondek M, Themann H, Nieschlag E (1987a) Hypogonadotropic status and testicular morphology in nonhuman primates (Macaca mulatta and M fascicularis). In: Spera G, de Kretser DM (eds) Morphological basis of human reproductive function. Plenum, New York, pp 45–48

Weinbauer GF, Respondek M, Themann H, Nieschlag E (1987b) Reversibility of long-term effects of GnRH agonist administration on testicular histology and sperm production in the nonhuman primate. J Androl 8:319–329

Weinbauer GF, Surmann FJ, Nieschlag E (1987c) Suppression of spermatogenesis in a nonhuman primate (Macaca fascicularis) by concomitant gonadotropin-releasing hormone antagonist and testosterone treatment. Acta Endocrinol (Copenh) 114:138–146

Weinbauer GF, Göckeler E, Nieschlag E (1988) Testosterone prevents complete suppression of spermatogenesis in the gonadotropin-releasing hormone (GnRH) antagonist-treated nonhuman primate (Macaca fascicularis). J Clin Endocrinol Metab 67:284–290

Weinbauer GF, Khurshid S, Fingscheidt U, Nieschlag E (1989) Sustained inhibition of sperm production and inhibin secretion induced by a gonadotrophin-releasing hormone antagonist and delayed testosterone substitution in nonhuman primates (Macaca fascicularis). J Endocrinol 123:303–310

Weinbauer GF, Behre HM, Nieschlag E (1990) Contraceptive studies with GnRH analogs in men and nonhuman primates. In: Bouchard P, Haour F, Franchimont P, Schatz B (eds) Recent progress on GnRH and gonadal peptides. Elsevier, Paris, pp 181–194

Weinbauer GF, Behre HM, Fingscheidt U, Nieschlag E (1991a) Human follicle-stimulating hormone exerts a stimulatory effect on spermatogenesis, testicular size, and serum inhibin levels in the gonadotropin-releasing hormone antagonist-treated nonhuman primate (Macaca fascicularis). Endocrinology 129:1831–1839

Weinbauer GF, Fingscheidt U, Khurshid S, Nieschlag E (1991b) Endocrine regulation of primate testicular function. In: Moudgal NR, Yoshinaga K, Rao AJ, Adiga PR (eds) Perspectives in primate reproductive biology. Wiley, New Delhi, pp 165–172

WHO: World Health Organization Task Force on Methods for the Regulation of Male Fertility (1990) Contraceptive efficacy of testosterone-induced azoospermia in normal men. Lancet 336:955–959

Wynn PC, Suarez-Quian CA, Childs GV, Catt KJ (1986) Pituitary binding and internalization of radioiodinated gonadotropin-releasing hormone agonist and antagonist ligands in vitro and in vivo. Endocrinology 119:1852–1863

Zarate A, Canales ES, Sthory I, Coy DH, Comaru-Schally AM, Schally AV (1981) Anovulatory effect of a LH-RH antagonist in women. Contraception 24:315–320

Subject Index